Public Health in India

Despite rapid advances in modern medicine and state-of-the-art healthcare services in the private sector, primary healthcare in India remains inaccessible to a majority of the population; even policy makers do not often have access to real-time data to fine-tune their policies or design appropriate research and intervention programmes.

Drawing on field experiences, this volume brings together scholars and practitioners to examine public health from different perspectives. It discusses practical and applied issues related to the health sector, especially the role of information and communications technology (ICT); participation of civil society; service delivery; quality evaluation; consumer empowerment; data management; and research and intervention.

This book will be useful to scholars, students and practitioners of public health in developing countries such as India. It will also interest policy makers, healthcare professionals, departments of public health management and those concerned with community medicine.

Diatha Krishna Sundar is Professor of Operations Management; Chairperson of Production & Operations Management Area; and Chairperson — ERP Center, Indian Institute of Management Bangalore (IIMB).

Shashank Garg is Chief Executive Officer of Handheld Solutions & Research Labs (HANDSREL), Bangalore.

Isha Garg is a Medical Doctor and was Professor of Pathology, and a former head, at St. John's Medical College, Bangalore.

Public Health in India

*Technology, governance
and service delivery*

EDITED BY

Diatha Krishna Sundar,
Shashank Garg and
Isha Garg

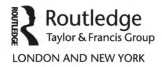

Routledge
Taylor & Francis Group

LONDON AND NEW YORK

First published 2015 by Routledge

2 Park Square, Milton Park, Abingdon, Oxfordshire OX14 4RN
711 Third Avenue, New York, NY 10017

Routledge is an imprint of the Taylor & Francis Group, an informa business

First issued in paperback 2017

British Library Cataloguing-in-Publication Data
A catalogue record for this book is available from the British Library

Library of Congress Cataloging-in-Publication Data
A catalog record has been requested for this book

ISBN: 978-1-138-89839-4 (hbk)
ISBN: 978-0-8153-7333-9 (pbk)

Typeset in Sabon 10/12pt by Glyph Graphics Private Limited Delhi 110 096

Contents

Figures

Tables

Abbreviations

AIIMS	All India Institute of Medical Sciences
ANC	anti-natal care
ASHA	A Source of Hope for All
CBO	community-based organisations
CDC	Centers for Disease Control
CHC	community health centre
CIH	Community Involvement in Health
CRF	case report form
DARPG	Department of Administrative Reforms and Public Grievances
DOTS	Directly Observed Treatment, Short-Course
EDC	electronic data capture
EMR	electronic medical record
FDA	Food and Drug Administration
FHIMS	Family Welfare and Health Information Monitoring System
GIS	geographical information system
GPHIN	Global Public Health Intelligence Network
GPRS	General Packet Radio Service
GPS	global positioning system
GUI	graphical user interface
HCP	healthcare professional
HIPAA	Health Insurance Portability and Accountability Act
HIS	Healthcare Information Systems
HSB	high-speed broadband
IATV	interactive television
ICT	information and communication technologies
ICU	intensive care unit
IDSP	Integrated Disease Surveillance Programme
IHC	India Healthcare
IP	Internet Protocol
IRB	Institutional Review Board
IT	information technology
MTP	medical termination of pregnancy

NAMI	Nodal Association on Mental Illness
NASSCOM	National Association of Software and Services Companies
NCD	non-communicable disease
NCR	National Capital Region
NGO	non-governmental organisation
NIMHANS	National Institute of Mental Health and Neurosciences
OSS	open-source software
OTTET	Orissa Trust of Technical Education and Training
PA	physician assistant
PAIS	process-aware information systems
PCPNDT	Pre-conception and Pre-natal Diagnostic Techniques (Act)
PDA	personal digital assistant
RA	research assistant
RNTCP	Revised National TB Control Programme
SARS	Severe Acute Respiratory Syndrome
SMS	short message service
SST	self-service technology
STBMI	School of Telemedicine and Biomedical Informatics
SWOT	strengths, weaknesses, opportunities, threats
TB	tuberculosis
UI	user interface
UN	United Nations
USG	ultrasonography
VBP	values-based practice
VoIP	Voice over Internet Protocol
WFMS	workflow management systems
WHO	World Health Organization

Contributors

Manigrib Bag is a senior faculty member at the Institute of Business Management and Research, Nodal Centre of West Bengal University of Technology. He teaches mainly in the areas of marketing, systems management and business law. He has post-graduate degrees in marine science and business management, as well as an MPhil degree in management. He is also a qualified law graduate. He publishes regularly in prominent journals, and also undertakes corporate consultancy.

Arunabha Biswas works as a consultant at Price waterhouse Coopers, primarily in the area of e-governance. He has experience in the domains of AS IS, business process re-engineering, and requests for proposal preparation, among other areas. He has worked on several key projects in the government sector. Prior to becoming a consultant, he was involved with implementation projects and application development for Tata Consultancy Services. An electronics engineer, he holds a postgraduate diploma in management from the T. A. Pai Management Institute, Manipal, with specialisation in marketing and IT.

Repu Daman Chand currently works on designing, operating and supporting the telemedicine technical network of the Sanjay Gandhi Post Graduate Institute of Medical Sciences (SGPGI), Lucknow. He is also a participant in the National Medical College Network Project at the National Resource Center, School of Telemedicine and Biomedical Informatics (STBMI), SGPGI, a project supported by the Ministry of Health and Family Welfare, Government of India. He was earlier involved in international projects like the WHO–DPR Korea Telemedicine Project in 2008 and the IHDP–World Bank Project in 2008 for establishing telemedicine networks.

Weiqin Chen is Professor at the Department of Information Science and Media Studies, University of Bergen, Norway. She received her PhD in Computer Science from the Chinese Academy of Sciences. She has participated in a number of national and international projects, including the OMEVAC projects funded by the Norwegian Research Council. Currently, her research focuses on mobile health information systems and technology-enhanced collaborative learning and work.

Laxmikant Deshmukh is currently Managing Director, Maharashtra Film, Stage and Cultural Development Corporation, Mumbai. An IAS officer, he initiated the Save the Baby Girl campaign in Kolhapur district of Maharashtra in 2009 during his tenure as Collector. He is also the author of many short stories and novels, and has won various literary awards.

P. Ganesan is Senior Professor of Marketing, VIT Business School, VIT University, Tamil Nadu. He has coedited two books in the areas of services and development economics, and has published over 60 research articles in reputed national and international journals. He has also presented numerous research papers at reputed national and international conferences. His current research involves the areas of inter–intra firm analysis, choice analysis in service products, and brand and service innovation.

Qian Gao completed her PhD from the College of Pharmacy, University of South Carolina. Her doctoral research sought to determine the chemopreventive effect of dietary phytochemicals on carcinogen-induced lung cancer, and to understand the molecular mechanism through which certain phytochemicals modulate lung cancer progression. In 2006, she enrolled in an MS programme in the clinical research methods track of biostatistics. She has been an associate member of the American Association of Cancer Research since 2004, and is also a certified SAS base programmer.

Isha Garg is Professor of Pathology at St. John's Medical College, Bengaluru. She was a Fellow in the Reuters Digital Vision Program at Stanford University in 2006–07, during which period she worked on a project to develop a mobile technology framework for disease surveillance. Professor Garg has a keen interest in the application of ICT technologies in the practice of medicine and public health. She has published extensively in peer-reviewed national and international journals and presented papers at several conferences.

Shashank Garg is CEO of Handheld Solutions & Research Labs (HANDSREL), a Bangalore-based company developing advanced mobile solutions for improvements in service delivery in the area of public health. He is also an active founder-member of the OpenXdata Consortium. He was a co-inventor of the Simputer, a low-cost, mobile computing device developed with the goal of applying appropriate technologies for bridging the digital divide in developing countries. Dr Garg has contributed several articles in international peer-reviewed journals, international conference proceedings, and edited book chapters.

Stan Kachnowski is a leading scholar of healthcare information policy and management, and has taught e-health and healthcare e-business for nearly 20 years. He has authored over 100 scholarly papers and presentations in healthcare technology management, informatics and e-governance. In 1996 he was elected to the US-based College of Healthcare Information Management Executives. In 2003, he was elected a Fellow of the Royal Society of Medicine, UK, for his research with the National Health Service in using handhelds to track patient data. He is currently Visiting Professor at the Indian Institute of Technology Delhi, while also overseeing all programmatic activities at HITLAB.

Elise Kang is Research Coordinator at Healthcare Innovation and Technology Lab (HITLAB), New York. She previously worked as a research assistant at the Laboratory of Cognitive Neurscience, Boston Children's Hospital. She is currently pursuing her MD at Case Western Reserve University School of Medicine.

Jørn Klungsøyr is a PhD Fellow at the Centre for International Health, University of Bergen. His focus over the past decade has been on developing open-source technologies and collaborations for mobile data capture and management in low-resource settings (http://www.openxdata.org). He has been co-leading the research projects mVAC for mobile vaccination registries and OMEVAC for mobile data capture in clinical trials funded by the Norwegian Research Council.

Diatha Krishna Sundar is Professor of Operations Management, Chairperson of Production & Operations Management Area, and also Chairperson, ERP Center, at the Indian Institute of Management Bangalore. Prior to this, he served as a faculty member at the Indian Institute of Technology Kharagpur. Professor Krishna Sundar has 18 years of research and teaching experience. His areas of research include IT strategy, e-business management, e-governance, operations strategy, enterprise resource planning, supply chain management and manufacturing strategy. Professor Sundar is a consultant to many manufacturing & service (IT) organizations as well as government departments, both in India and abroad, in the areas of operations strategy, supply-chain management, IT strategy, e-governance and ERP implementation. He has published more than 70 research articles in international journals, international conference proceedings and book chapters.

J. Ajith Kumar is Professor and Associate Dean (Research) at the T. A. Pai Management Institute (TAPMI), Manipal, in the area of operations management. At TAPMI, he teaches courses on operations research, simulation modelling, system dynamics and game theory. Professor Ajith Kumar holds BTech and MTech degrees, both from the Indian Institute of Technology Kanpur, and a PhD from the Indian Institute of Technology Madras. He had nearly 12 years of industry experience prior to his stint in academia.

Girish Lad is Chairman and Managing Director of Magnum Opus IT Consulting, a firm that focuses on innovations that help achieve transparent governance. He is the inventor of a system for the effective implementation of the PCPNDT Act, popularly known as the Active Tracker, which was successfully used in the Save the Baby Girl campaign. Girish Lad's various innovations have earned him the prestigious Times of India Social Impact Award, the Manthan Award, the NASSCOM Foundation Award, the eIndia Award, and the Rajiv Gandhi Maharashtra Information Technology Award for e-governance.

R. Lakshmi is a doctoral student at VIT University. Her research focuses mainly on the dynamics that exist between individuals and technology, especially self-service technology interfaces, with the aim of throwing light on emergent behaviours that remain insufficiently explained by existing theories. She has more than six years of industrial experience in the services sector.

Saroj Kanta Mishra is Professor and Head of the Department of Endocrine Surgery at Sanjay Gandhi Post Graduate Institute of Medical Sciences (SGPGI), Lucknow. He was instrumental in establishing the Telemedicine Society of India at Lucknow in 2001. He was also instrumental in setting up the School of Telemedicine and Biomedical Informatics at SGPGI, now recognised as a National Resource Center for Telemedicine and Biomedical Informatics by the Government of India. He has served as an e-health and telemedicine expert for the International Telecommunication Union, the World Health Organization (WHO) and other international agencies. He was recently nominated a member of the e-Health Technical Advisory Group, WHO.

Raghu K. Mittal is Co-founder and Technical Lead of Handheld Solutions Research Labs (HANDSREL). He is an active contributor to OpenXdata, an open-source consortium for mobile data collection. He is one of the four core-committers at the group, with committing rights to the main OpenXdata repository. He has also worked on creating a tool called OpenXanalyzer, a GUI-based analysis tool based on R. He presented a paper on the viability of R as an analysis tool at the International Congress of E-government in 2010.

Aritra Pal is a business consultant at Cognizant Business Consulting. He has worked on numerous projects involving programme management, strategy consulting, DPR preparation, business process re-engineering, assessment and evaluation, among other areas. Key among these projects have been the State eGov Mission Projects, Tea Board of India, ePRI and e-District. Aritra Pal holds a postgraduate diploma in management from the T. A. Pai Management Institute. He has strong research interests in e-governance and has attended various national and international e-governance seminars.

Candice D. Presseau is a doctoral student at the College of Education, Lehigh University. She earlier worked for HITLAB as a research associate, and also completed a year-long internship at the Center for Family Connections in Cambridge, Massachusetts, where she provided therapeutic services to children and families affected by issues of adoption and foster care. She has an MA in counselling psychology from Boston College and an MA in quantitative methods in the social sciences from Columbia University.

Chhanda Ray is Associate Professor at the RCC Institute of Information Technology, Kolkata. She completed her Phd in Computer Science & Engineering from Jadavpur University, Kolkata, and has more than 20 publications in different international journals and conferences in the areas of distributed system, image processing, data mining and public health. Her book *Distributed Database Systems* was published in 2009.

Maheswar Satpathy is a trained clinical psychologist with training experience in the areas of neuropsychology and mental health assessment. He is currently working on his PhD at the University of New South Wales, Sydney, as an Australian Leadership Awards Scholar (final phase) in the area of interdisciplinary public health. His research focuses on risk behaviours which may lead to HIV/AIDS and STIs among young and vulnerable sexual minority populations in developing country contexts like South Asia, more specifically India.

Osman R. Sayan specialises in emergency medicine and internal medicine, and has been practising for over 27 years. He currently practises in New York, New York. Dr Sayan completed medical school at Rutgers Robert Wood Johnson Medical School, and is licensed to treat patients in New York and New Jersey.

Indra Pratap Singh is a Telemedicine Project Manager at the School of Telemedicine and Biomedical Informatics (STBMI), Sanjay Gandhi Post Graduate Institute of Medical Sciences, Lucknow. He is also closely associated with training and diploma courses at STBMI, and serves in the capacity of Training Coordinator. He has a master's degree in bioinformatics from Allahabad Agricultural Institute. Indra Pratap Singh has played a key role in the development of the low-cost, portable mHealth toolkit and mobile telemedicine system.

Peter Wakholi is Lecturer at the School of Computing and Informatics Technology at Makerere University. He received his PhD at the University of Bergen, Norway. His doctoral research focused on process-aware mobile systems. He has implemented his research on workflows through the OpenXdata mobile data collection platform. Currently, he is pursuing research in e-health systems.

Introduction

Issues, Challenges and the Role of Technology

◼

The success of any society can be measured on the basis of the three critical attributes of health, education and financial activity. These attributes form a three-legged stool that is stable only if each leg is equal to the other two in length. Communities will feel empowered and be lifted out of poverty only if they have access to good health, good primary, secondary and higher education, and finance to pursue economic activity. The task of a good political system is to provide healthy, progressive and stable governance structures which can focus on delivering healthcare and education and facilitate equitable economic opportunity for all citizens cost-effectively. In this book, we focus on the importance of public health in a healthy society, and on the role of technology in the dissemination of these services even to citizens in remote locations. We begin by introducing a commonly accepted definition of 'public health', and familiarising the reader with the concept of disease surveillance.

Public Health and Its Importance

The concept of 'public health', as distinguished from the practice of modern medicine, is not sufficiently understood beyond the circles of practising professionals and experts in the field. Even among healthcare professionals, public health is often erroneously treated as an extension of community medicine. Public health is taught as a graduate-level specialisation in very few medical colleges in India. In order to establish an appropriate context for this book, it is important to understand the basic concept of public health and highlight the differences between public health and healthcare.

Modern healthcare has made rapid advances in the diagnosis and treatment of major diseases, with the evolution of a high degree of super-specialisation and personalised treatment. However, the healthcare system has not demonstrated improved health outcomes.

In the last few decades, excellent tertiary-care facilities have become available even in developing countries like India, but there is little empirical evidence to suggest whether these facilities are affordable and equitably accessible for the average citizen. It is clear that the cost of diagnostic services, hospitalisation, treatment, drugs and professional fees has increased without bound, whereas the benefits of medicine have not percolated down to the average citizen. Unfortunately, modern healthcare does not focus on the social and economic aspects of disease. It is estimated that over 70 per cent of the Indian population is still considered medically under-served, despite the country having embraced modern healthcare practices for decades.

So, what is public health? Public health is often defined as 'the science and art of preventing disease, prolonging life and promoting health through organised societal efforts', encouraging the use of social policy as a tool for engaging communities in the prevention of disease (Alderslade 1990). The primary healthcare system, along with disease surveillance (which will be discussed shortly), is the most important tool in the hands of public health officials. Epidemiological studies provide insights into factors that cause diseases which might be preventable, and enhance our understanding of the prevention techniques required for improving health outcomes. In other words, public health deals with the health of communities and large populations, which may involve education, lifestyle and behaviour modification, research into the preventive aspects of disease and injury, as well as research into the social impact and economic burden of diseases. Focus on prevention rather than on treatment is the cornerstone of public health programmes, and it is an important tool in the global fight against disease.

Disease Surveillance Systems

Primary healthcare services play an essential role in a vibrant public health system. However, the public health system must also use have the capacity to continually monitor potential threats and isolate them in real time. Disease surveillance is a basic tool of the field epidemiologist. Surveillance data provide a scientific basis for an appropriate healthcare policy, disease control decisions, evaluation of efforts, and allocation of resources in primary healthcare. Thacker and Birkhead (2002: 27) provide the following well-accepted definition of surveillance in public health practice which is promoted by the Centers for Disease Control (CDC, Atlanta, USA):

> Public health surveillance (sometimes called epidemiological surveillance) is the ongoing systematic collection, analysis, and interpretation of outcome-specific data essential to the planning, implementation and evaluation of public health practice, closely integrated with the timely dissemination of this data to those who need to know. Outcomes may include disease, injury, and disability, as well as risk factors, vector exposures, environmental hazards, or other exposures. The final link of the surveillance chain is the application of these data to prevent and control human disease and injury.

Disease surveillance, which is an important aspect of any public healthcare programme, serves two essential purposes: (*a*) monitoring the progress of ongoing medical interventions for disease reduction; and (*b*) early detection of outbreaks to initiate investigative and control measures (John 2002; John, Rajappan et al. 2004). Surveillance in the public health system serves as an early warning system to detect, diagnose and monitor impending health hazards in the community. Global disease surveillance systems such as the Global Public Health Intelligence Network (GPHIN),[1] developed in the Canadian public health system in collaboration with the World Health Organization (WHO), have proved useful in early detection and containment in the major Severe Acute Respiratory Syndrome (SARS) epidemic that was first detected in China in 2003. The avian flu which followed the SARS epidemic was even more serious, and could potentially have resulted in major health disasters of pandemic proportions if not detected early.

Thomas (2002) and Heymann (2004) describe the state of the disease surveillance system prevailing in India. Early work on the Vellore model of disease surveillance is described by John, Samuel et al. (1998), John (2002) and John, Rajappan et al. (2004). A district-level model of disease surveillance was developed in conformance with the Vellore model and first demonstrated in North Arcot district of Tamil Nadu (south India). It was subsequently piloted in another district of Kerala (John, Rajappan et al. 2004). For further insight into disease surveillance, see Buehler (1998), Cheung (2003) and Thacker and Birkhead (2002).

India has had an Integrated Disease Surveillance Programme (IDSP) in place since 2004, which collects raw data from a large number of sources in primary healthcare centres across the country. But the programme has not sufficiently embraced mobile computing and communications technologies, and is therefore unable to function as a sentinel outbreak detection programme, as was initially intended. Outbreaks generally occur due to very specific local conditions, but remain undetected because of lack of awareness and expertise at the local level. Healthcare professionals and local governments recognise the value of early detection of the onset of epidemics for appropriate intervention and containment measures. But they have not used modern technology effectively. India's IDSP collects raw data on 14 infectious or communicable diseases based on syndromic definitions, but non-communicable diseases (NCDs), also known as 'lifestyle diseases', are also becoming a major cause of concern to public health professionals. Thus, robust surveillance systems must also cater to NCDs with a high level of attention.

The Case for TB Surveillance

Tuberculosis (TB) is a major global health problem. It is estimated that in 2012, about 8.6 million people developed TB, and around 1.3 million died from the disease. The number of TB deaths is unacceptably large, given that most cases are preventable if detected and treated early (WHO 2013). Southeast Asia and the Western Pacific together account for almost 58 per cent of detected cases. India accounts for almost 26 per cent of globally detected cases, while China accounts for close to 12 per cent of globally detected cases. While the TB mortality rate has been reduced by 45 per cent since 1992, the WHO's target is to reduce deaths by 50 per cent by 2015. Tuberculosis is a highly infectious disease which spreads primarily through the air from a person suffering from TB. A single patient is estimated to infect 10 or more people in a year due to close association within a family environment (RNTCP 2001, 2002, 2013).

In India, according to estimates published on the official website of TB Control in India, an organisation under the Ministry of Health and Family Welfare, over 1.8 million persons develop the disease every year, of which about 800,000 cases are infectious. Until recently, 370,000 died of TB annually (RNTCP 2001, 2002, 2013, 2014). The disease poses a major barrier to social and economic development, since an estimated 100 million workdays are lost due to illness. The national economic burden due to TB is estimated to be in excess of US$3 billion in indirect costs, and around US$300 million in direct costs. Though most deaths due to TB occur among men, the burden of TB is higher on women. In India, TB is the cause of the second largest number of deaths from any disease. Hence, with the staggering burden of TB and the human suffering it causes, controlling TB in India is a major challenge for the public health system.

The WHO has recommended a strategy to control TB, known as Directly Observed Treatment, Short-Course (DOTS). India started its National Tuberculosis Programme in 1992, and then reintroduced an improved programme called the Revised National TB Control Programme (RNTCP) in 1993 based on the DOTS recommendations. It has been observed that the majority of patients in developing countries with high TB incidence are not treated under DOTS (WHO 2002, 2013). Instead, these patients are treated by private providers who are not formally involved in the RNTCP system. Private practitioners usually do not notify detected cases, and rarely use recommended TB case management principles, which results in poor treatment outcomes (Lonnroth 2000; Uplekar and Pathania 2001; Uplekar et al. 2001). Involvement of private practitioners in RNTCP has been recommended as a means to increase the proportion of patients treated under DOTS. To improve the case detection rate, a number of steps, such as notification of detected cases, have been made mandatory.

The economic burden posed by TB, and India's status as a major contributor to the incidence of TB, make it imperative that TB surveillance is treated as a priority public health problem. Research has shown that when detected early, TB is completely curable, provided the patient completes the full course of treatment without interruptions. Adherence to treatment is a major problem that may be solved through the deployment of mobile technology for monitoring adherence.

A Rationale for Mobile Communications

Is there a rationale for using mobile technology in disease surveillance and public health? Data from the annual reports published by the Telecom Regulatory Authority of India, presented in Table 0.1, shows a telephony subscriber base in excess of 850 million subscribers, with a decline in wire-line subscribers and an explosive increase in wireless subscribers (TRAI 2007, 2008, 2009, 2010, 2011, 2012, 2013).

Table 0.1 Data on Telecom Subscribers in India

	Financial Year (from 1 April to 31 March)					
	2007–08	*2008–09*	*2009–10*	*2010–11*	*2011–12*	*2012–13*
Wire-line subscribers (millions)	39.42	37.96	36.96	34.73	32.17	30.21
Wireless subscribers (millions)	261.07	391.76	584.32	811.59	919.17	867.8
Broadband subscribers (millions)		6.22	8.77	11.89	13.81	15.05
Subscribers added per month (millions)	8	10	15	18.9		4.02
Rural tele-density (%)	9.2	15.2	24.29	33.79	39.22	40.23
Overall tele-density (%)	26.22	36.98	52.74	70.89	78.66	70.85

Source: TRAI (2007, 2008, 2009, 2010, 2011, 2012, 2013).

Figure 0.1 shows the steady growth of rural tele-density in India over the same period. Nationwide tele-density has saturated and is experiencing some decline, whereas rural tele-density is approaching saturation at a lower rate. With the simultaneous growth in mobile broadband access, mobile telephony is transitioning from voice-based services to embracing voice and data simultaneously. The next level of growth will probably be fuelled by lower pricing due to competitive pressures, faster data speeds and compelling data-oriented services. Can public health policy makers and stakeholders afford to miss out on the mobile revolution? With India now contributing over 13 per cent of the world's 6.5 billion mobile subscribers, there is a clear rationale for application providers to leverage the mobile communication infrastructure with user-centric applications.

Communication costs have already come down in India and are among the lowest in the world. The country is undergoing a transition from pure voice telephony to data communications, as communication speeds transition from 2G (GPRS/EDGE technologies) to 3G, 4G and beyond. Thus, the growth and reach of the cellular communications infrastructure present a unique opportunity for

Figure 0.1 Growth of Rural Tele-density in India

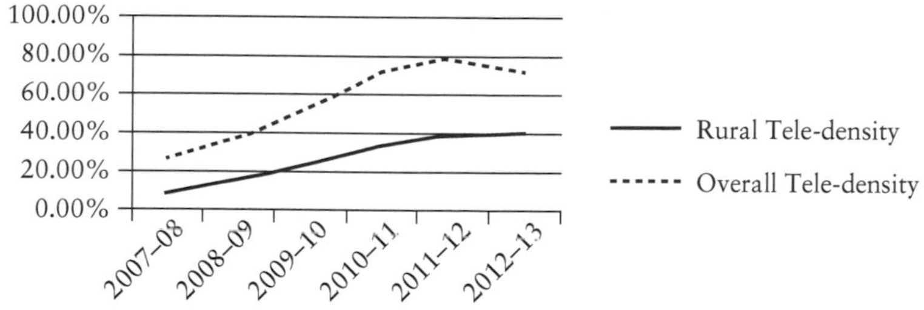

Source: TRAI (2007, 2008, 2009, 2010, 2011, 2012, 2013).

developing mobile computing and communications infrastructure for large-scale deployment of mobile applications. While the first generation of mobile applications were relatively simple, based largely on short messaging services and limited in functionality, the current generation of mobile applications use bi-directional voice and data communication to present a highly interactive interface that can handle complex forms, transfer information from the mobile phone to a remote server, and receive a response in real time. In addition, back-end services are hosted in the cloud, which makes it easier to scale cost-effectively. The next generation of mobile applications will use higher bandwidths provided by the communication infrastructure to embrace multiple media streams and present virtual reality interfaces to their users.

It is in this context that healthcare policy makers must look at improving public health services relating to disease prevention through better education and dissemination of information on health and hygiene, disease surveillance, and data collection and analysis in real time. Information and communication technologies (ICT), particularly with the rapid proliferation of mobile communications, will play an enabling role in better delivery of primary healthcare services and in increasing coverage to remote, medically under-served communities. However, public health and healthcare professionals are generally averse to technology adoption unless that technology is directly relevant to diagnostics. At the same time, technology professionals lack the domain knowledge required to understand use-case scenarios in public health space. This gap can be filled by bringing together professionals from diverse backgrounds on a common platform for the exchange of information and experience. The objective of this volume on public health is to attempt to bridge that gap between public health professionals and technology providers by presenting some practical cases of work done at the intersection of public health and technology. The editors use a broader definition of public health than the one provided earlier to enable inclusion of the work being done in the primary healthcare system.

The first chapter, titled 'Save the Baby Girl', by Girish Lad and Laxmikant Deshmukh, presents an example of how modern technologies are often applied in socially unacceptable ways, in this case for the determination of the sex of an unborn child, leading to the termination of pregnancy if a girl is detected. This represents an extreme example of the unintended consequences of technology deployment, and holds up a mirror to us as a society. The gender ratio is tilting adversely against the girl child, resulting in long-term social consequences that can only be imagined. This case study represents a classic case for inclusion in a book on public health. The authors have developed a monitor that can be attached to the sonograph machine. Their case study demonstrates how the deviant behaviour of doctors and technicians can be monitored and reported to reduce the incidence of sex determination. Of course, long-term studies need to be done before we can conclude whether such techniques result in improved outcomes.

In the second chapter, Candice D. Presseau, Qian Gao, Osman R. Sayan, Elise Kang and Stan Kachnowski present a study on communication trends among hospital personnel in multi-site environments. This work is based on a research study conducted in four New York hospitals. While it could be said that the link to public health is a bit tenuous, we have chosen to include this chapter as it addresses critical issues in communication between healthcare personnel operating in multi-site environments, a situation that often prevails in the primary healthcare sector.

In the third chapter, Chhanda Ray and Manigrib Bag describe their work on measurements of service quality in the healthcare sector, based on a model that incorporates seven qualitative parameters including tangibles, assurance, responsiveness, reliability, empathy, image and technical quality. Without a high degree of customer satisfaction, positive public health outcomes may be difficult to achieve. So the primary healthcare system also needs to define its own service quality measures, and make periodic assessments of customer satisfaction to determine whether intended outcomes have been attained or not.

In Chapter 4, Aritra Pal, Arunabha Biswas and J. Ajith Kumar present findings from a study on the potential challenges that an e-government project in the public health domain could face. They classify these challenges into the different categories of technological, socio-economic, human resource, operational and strategic challenges, and develop a framework of interactions between the different categories of challenges. The authors suggest that this framework of interactions between challenges could be a useful tool in assessing the risks involved in such a project. As e-governance projects are inherently technology-oriented, it is important to understand whether these projects are sustainable despite the many challenges they may face. This would also be useful in the governance of other public health projects which often involve a diverse range of challenges.

In the fifth chapter, Maheswar Satpathy describes how non-governmental organisations (NGOs) can leverage ICT for the promotion of community-based mental healthcare. Mental health is another major problem in the public health space. Satpathy suggests that the role of NGOs, because they tend to focus on learning by doing, is particularly relevant in engaging communities in social causes.

In Chapter 6, Raghu Mittal describes how certain open-source tools could be deployed as viable alternatives to proprietary, commercially available tools for statistical research in public health. Since researchers and practitioners in public health rely extensively on statistical analysis to identify trends and measure outcomes, open-source statistical analysis tools like 'R' must become an important part of their portfolio of tools, especially in the context of the low budgets generally available to researchers in public health.

In the seventh chapter, Repu Daman Chand, Indra Pratap Singh and Saroj Kanta Mishra describe a mobile, telemedicine solution that has been developed for the delivery of healthcare services in rural and remote communities. They present a practical case study of this application in a rural setting. In Chapter 8, R. Lakshmi and P. Ganesan study whether the use of self-service technologies in telemedicine facilitates the empowerment of customers, enhances customer involvement in healthcare, and provides a better overall customer experience.

In the ninth chapter, Peter Wakholi, Weiqin Chen and Jørn Klungsøyr of the University of Bergen's Center for International Health provide a comprehensive framework for a mobile-phone-based electronic data capture (EDC) solution, with emphasis on a process orientation, for field data collection in clinical trials. Their framework uses workflow technologies to manage the specified process flows in a disconnected environment.

In the concluding chapter, Diatha Krishna Sundar, Shashank Garg and Isha Garg and present a mobile EDC system that has been developed under their supervision for applications in the public health domain. Public health researchers often use traditional pen-and-paper-based systems for field data collection, resulting in unreliable data, long lead times, lack of scalability, and difficulty in follow-up of cohorts in longitudinal studies. It is well known that the cost of correcting errors increases as data moves further away from the source of input. Mobile EDC systems can overcome a lot of these problems by reducing the chance of errors, as data is captured at its source. The authors present one such system that has been developed and deployed in many public health research projects and even in e-governance.

Many people have been involved in the preparation of content for this book, besides the authors who agreed to contribute chapters for this initiative. Initial contributions to editing were made by Mrs Sarita Deshpande, who was earlier at IIM Bangalore. The publisher's editing team spent many months editing the papers and interfacing with the authors for improving their manuscripts, and interfacing with the editors to ensure that the book saw the light of day. In a publishing endeavour that spans a few years, the state of the practice does not stay stagnant. The editors have tried to ensure that the topics chosen remain relevant to the original goal of bridging the gap between public health and technology. This task was well coordinated by Ms Shoma Choudhury, with the able assistance of Ms Antara Ray Chaudhury, Ms. Rimina Mohapatra, Ms. Aruna Ramachandran and Ms. Denise File on behalf of the publishing team. The editors are thankful to all these people who have contributed to the eventual publication of this volume. Errors and inaccuracies, if any, are the collective responsibility of the editors.

Note

1. For more information on GPHIN, see World Health Organization, Global Alert and Response (GAR), 'Epidemic Intelligence: Systematic Event

Detection', http://www.who.int/csr/alertresponse/epidemicintelligence/
en/ (accessed on 23 December 2014).

References

Alderslade, R. (1990). 'Public Health Management in the Health-for-All Era', *World Health Forum*, vol. 11, pp. 269–73.

Buehler, J. (1998). 'Surveillance', in *Modern Epidemiology* (2nd edn), edited by K. J. Rothman and S. Greenland, Philadelphia: Lippincott-Raven Publishers, pp. 435–57.

Cheung, S. (2003). 'White Paper: The IT Infrastructure of Hong Kong's Centre for Disease Control (CDC)', DO IT Think Tank, Hong Kong.

Heymann, D. L. (2004). 'From Smallpox to Polio and Beyond: Disease Surveillance in India', *Indian Journal of Medical Research*, vol. 120, pp. 70–72.

John, T. J. (2002). 'Disease Surveillance for Disease Control: The Vellore Model', *Christian Medical College Alumni Journal*, vol. 36, pp. 13–17.

John, T. J., K. Rajappan and K. K. Arjunan (2004). 'Communicable Diseases Monitored by Disease Surveillance in Kottayam District, Kerala State, India', *Indian Journal of Medical Research*, vol. 120, pp. 86–93.

John, T. J., R. Samuel, V. Balraj and R. John (1998). 'Disease Surveillance at District Level: A Model for Developing Countries', *Lancet*, vol. 352, pp. 58–61.

Lonnroth, K. (2000). 'Public Health in Private Hands: Studies on Private and Public Tuberculosis Cure in Ho Chi Minh City, Vietnam', PhD thesis, University of Gothenberg.

RNTCP (Revised National TB Control Programme) (2001). 'Revised National Tuberculosis Control Programme's Operational Guidelines for Tuberculosis Control', Directorate General of Health Services, New Delhi.

——— (2002). *TB India 2002: Revised National Tuberculosis Control Programme Annual Report*, Directorate General of Health Services, New Delhi, http://tbcindia.nic.in/documents.html (accessed on 15 February 2015).

——— (2013). *TB India 2013: Revised National Tuberculosis Control Programme Annual Report*, Directorate General of Health Services, New Delhi, http://www.tbcindia.nic.in/pdfs/tb%20india%202013.pdf (accessed on 15 February 2015).

——— (2014). *TB India 2014: Revised National Tuberculosis Control Programme Annual Report*, Directorate General of Health Services, New Delhi, http://www.tbcindia.nic.in/pdfs/TB%20INDIA%202014.pdf (accessed on 15 February 2015).

Thacker, S. B., and G. S. Birkhead (2002). 'Surveillance', in *Field Epidemiology* (2nd edn), edited by M. B. Gregg, New York: Oxford University Press, pp. 27–50.

Thomas, K. (2002). 'Integrated Disease Surveillance Program: A Priority Health Program for the Country', *CMC Research Bulletin*, vol. 21, pp. 2–5.

TRAI (Telecom Regulatory Authority of India) (2007). *Annual Report 2006–07*, New Delhi: TRAI.

——— (2008). *Annual Report 2007–08*, New Delhi: TRAI.

——— (2009). *Annual Report 2008–09*, New Delhi: TRAI.

——— (2010). *Annual Report 2009–10*, New Delhi: TRAI.

——— (2011). *Annual Report 2010–11*, New Delhi: TRAI.

——— (2012). *Annual Report 2011–12*, New Delhi: TRAI.

——— (2013). *Annual Report 2012–13*, New Delhi: TRAI.

Uplekar, M., and V. Pathania (2001). 'Involving Private Practitioners in Tuberculosis Control: Issues, Interventions and Emerging Policy Framework', WHO/CDS/TB/2001.285, World Health Organization, Geneva.

Uplekar, M., V. Pathania and M. Raviglione (2001). 'Private Practitioners and Public Health: Weak Links in Tuberculosis Control', *Lancet*, vol. 385, pp. 912–16.

WHO (World Health Organization) (2002). 'Global Tuberculosis Control: Surveillance, Planning, Financing', WHO/CDs/TB 2002.29S, WHO, Geneva.

——— (2013). 'Global Tuberculosis Report 2013', WHO/HTM/TB/2013.11, WHO, Geneva.

1

Save the Baby Girl

Girish Lad and Laxmikant Deshmukh

◻

Misuse of the sonography machine in India has been the major reason for the steep decline in the sex ratio and the rise in illegal female foeticide across the nation. Sons are in huge demand in India due to various socio-economic factors. The government, even with strong legislation in the form of the Pre-conception and Pre-natal Diagnostic Techniques (PCPNDT) Act, has been unable to do much, since foeticide is carried out by doctors with the families' consent. The Save the Baby Girl initiative was launched when the 2001 census showed a sex ratio of 839 girls per 1,000 boys in Kolhapur district. The initiative addresses the two major issues of under-reporting and false reporting in cases of sex determination. An online portal was developed,[1] and 252 genetic centres started submitting sonography reports of pregnant females (form F), delivery reports, and medical termination of pregnancy (MTP) reports within 24 hours. However, the under-reporting problem was yet to be solved. A device called the 'Active Tracker' (its former version was known as the 'Silent Observer') was developed for this purpose. This device is attached to each sonography machine, and performs continuous screen capture of the machine monitor in the form of a video. The two-phase implementation of the Active Tracker has resulted in an increase in reporting by almost 50 per cent, as well as an increase in the sex ratio. As per the 2011 census, the sex ratio in Kolhapur district had gone up to 845, standing at 880 in September 2011.

Sex Selection and Female Foeticide

The United Nations Population Fund (UNFPA 2010) estimates that the practice of prenatal sex selection has resulted in approximately 600,000 girls being missed annually in India during the period 2001–07. This is roughly 1,600 girls per day. No state/union territory in India has a female child sex ratio over 1,000. Only 8 out of 35 states/union territories in India have had a positive female child sex ratio during the last 10 years. As Figure 1.1 shows, the sex ratio in India has been declining steadily in recent decades, from 945 in 1991, to 927 in 2001, and 914 in 2011. The reason for this dramatic decline stems from the introduction into India of methods of prenatal sex determination, such as amniocentesis and ultrasound technology. The emergence of sex identification techniques heralded a new discriminatory regime in India, which is responsible today for the dramatic sex ratio situation in many of the country's regions.

Figure 1.1 Sex Ratio Comparison

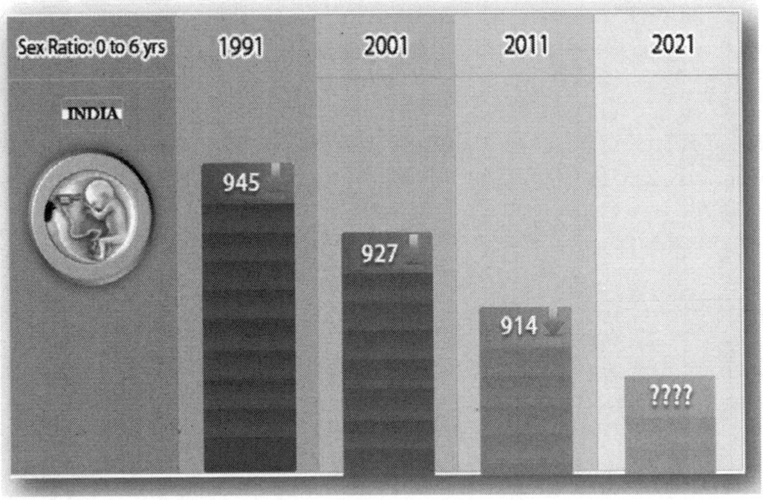

Source: Save the Baby Girl, http://www.savethebabygirl.org/images/STBG%20 Overview.pdf (accessed on 15 February 2015).

Sex selection in India does not take place in a legal vacuum. In fact, in 1983, just a few years after the introduction of the new ultrasound and amniocentesis technologies, the Indian Parliament banned the practice of sex determination in all public institutions. The prime legislation in this regard at the all-India level remains the Pre-Natal Diagnostic Techniques (Regulation and Prevention of Misuse) Act, passed in 1994 and later amended in 2003.

The law was primarily meant to address the issue of unwanted pregnancies, as part of a comprehensive family planning strategy that encompassed many contraceptive options as well. But the combination of new technologies for prenatal sex determination and abortion proved to be a dramatic cocktail, which would quickly become an efficient sex selection device. From the 1980s, sex selective abortions became the primary method used to alter the sex composition of children. The Pre-conception and Pre-natal Diagnostic Techniques (PCPNDT) Act provides formidable tools to act against the misuse of technology.

The PCPNDT Act

The PCPNDT Act passed by the Indian Parliament came into force in 1994 for the regulation and prevention of misuse of new diagnostic techniques. Subsequently, following a Supreme Court order on its proper implementation, certain amendments were made to the act. This revised act came into force in 1996. The act was amended again in 2003 to include pre-conception techniques.

According to the act, no person or technology, including a specialist or a team of specialists in the field of infertility, shall conduct or cause to be conducted, or aid in conducting by himself or by any other person, sex selection on a woman or a man or on both or on any tissue, embryo, concepts, fluid or gametes derived from either or both of them.

The PCPNDT Act, 1994, contains the following provisions:

1. It prohibits sex selection, both before and after conception (Section 3A of the act).
2. It regulates prenatal diagnostic techniques (e.g., amniocentesis and ultrasonography [USG]) for the detection of genetic abnormalities, by restricting their use to registered institutions.
3. The act allows the use of these techniques only at registered places for specified purposes and by qualified persons registered for this purpose (Section 4 of the act).
4. It provides for the prevention of misuse of such techniques of sex selection before or after conception (Section 6 of the act).
5. It prohibits the advertisement of any technique of sex selection as well as sex determination (Section 22 of the act).

6. It prohibits the sale of ultrasound machines to persons not registered under this act (Rule 3A, inserted vide GSR, 109[e], dt 14-2-2003).
7. It specifies punishments for violation of the provisions of the act (Section 23).

What's Going Wrong?

The enforcement of the PCPNDT Act, 2003, which prohibits sex determination tests on the foetus (leading to abortion in many cases if it is found to be a female), has been far from satisfactory. The main reasons for this have been:

1. poor supervision of genetic and ultrasound clinics
2. unethical and illegal practices by concerned doctors/ radiologists
3. rampant misuse of technology
4. fast increase in the number of ultrasound clinics over the years
5. poor implementation of the PCPNDT Act
6. failure of genetics centres to generate any records of illegal sex determination: there are no complainants and no evidence. Unfortunately, like many other acts, this act also faces implementation problems.
7. no effective monitoring mechanism
8. no proper knowledge of the law and procedures
9. no standardisation in practices, record keeping, etc.
10. problems of under-reporting and false reporting
11. failure to report critical records, as a result of which no proofs/evidence is available to authorities to take action

Solution: Save the Baby Girl and the Active Tracker

Stage I: Online Portal

A web portal, www.savethebabygirl.org, was developed as an online software solution that connects all genetics centres and collects important data on a daily basis as per PCPNDT Act rules and formats. The portal provides an electronic method of submission of data and reports to the appropriate government authorities.

The software ensures that incomplete data is not submitted by users. Government authorities can access this portal through a secure login, and can automatically generate various reports from time to time. The portal has all the features needed to carry out analysis of the data and generate pre-formatted statistical analysis reports, which can be leveraged for quick decision making and identification of problem areas.

The online portal helps the state by effectively implementing the PCPNDT Act. The solution covers all documentation facilities as per the act's provisions. It generates all the management information system reports that are required from time to time. The appropriate authorities can monitor state-level, district-level and block-level performance and carry out various activities such as centre applications, renewals and approvals.

The portal also offers the facility of generation of reports of action taken, details of court cases, machines sealed, etc. It has the following features:

1. data generation, auto-processing and analysis
2. collection of genetics centre data covering centres from both rural and urban areas, details of the centres' machines and employees, centre renewal reports, etc.
3. periodic (monthly) data reports for form F, delivery, MTP, rural-, urban- and district-level data comparison, etc.
4. data auto-analysis for suspected cases (i.e., women who have two or more girl children and have had a sonography done, women who are 35 years and above, abnormal deliveries, cases where MTP is advised, and abnormal sonography reports, among others)
5. age-wise patient analysis for the 0–18, 19–24, 25–34, and 35 years and above categories, data analysis of form F, delivery, MTP
6. pregnancy-related data analysis, such as trimester-wise data analysis, abnormal pregnancy reports, etc.
7. anti-natal care (ANC) tracking, area-wise ANC tracking through mobile-based short message service (SMS) reporting, missing cases, and analysis of all information which helps to formulate and fine-tune the implementation

The PCPNDT Compliance System for Genetic Centres has the following features:

1. secure login
2. daily submission of form F, delivery and MTP records
3. auto-generation of monthly reports
4. rejection of incomplete form Fs, enabling PCPNDT compliance
5. availability of support staff for documentation, as the online software is user-friendly
6. saving of time, effort and money in record keeping
7. no risk of sealing of action because of incomplete form Fs

Stage II: Active Tracker

Only the online portal was not enough, as it could not solve the problem of under-reporting and false reporting. To counter this problem, Magnum Opus invented a device called the 'Silent Observer'. An upgraded version, called 'Active Tracker' (Figure 1.2), was released later. This device is connected externally to the USG machine, and captures continuous video images of a working machine monitor.

Figure 1.2 Active Tracker

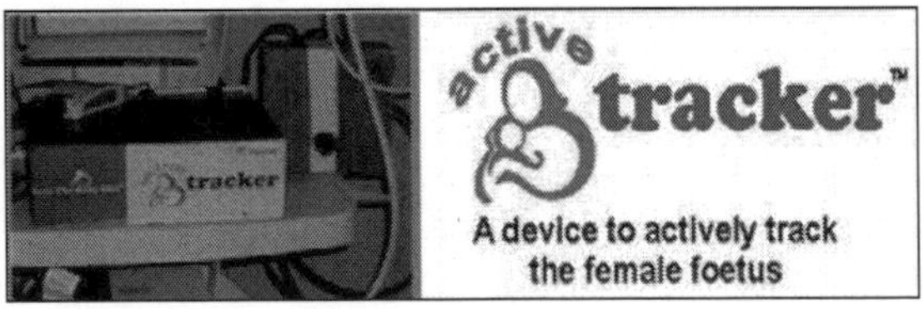

Source: Save the Baby Girl, http://www.savethebabygirl.org/images/STBG%20 Overview.pdf (accessed on 15 February 2015).

The Active Tracker is connected to the USG machine through external cables. The device has the following features:

1. The Active Tracker receives video signals from the USG machine. There is no interference with the USG machine, keeping the 'insurance' of the USG intact. No inputs are given to the USG machine.
2. The Active Tracker shares a common power supply with the USG machine, making the switching on or off of the Active Tracker and the USG machine simultaneous.

3. The Active Tracker has a storage capacity of 1 terabyte, which can be scaled up.
4. The video data is not uploaded to any server, but resides only on the Active Tracker.
5. To capture the data from the machine, appropriate authorisation is required. The transfer of data is secure.
6. The data is stored in an encrypted format, ensuring its security.

Some of the advanced features of the device include the following.

1. The Active Tracker has an inbuilt General Packet Radio Service (GPRS) facility through which every machine is connected to the portal www.savethebabygirl.org.
2. Each and every machine can be monitored remotely.
3. The device sends in alerts, e.g., when there is tampering with the machine, if unauthorised people try to access data, if the machine is switched off for more than 24 hours, etc.
4. The technology is foolproof, tamper-proof and highly secure.
5. It does not require any kind of sealing.

Kolhapur District: A Case Study

Background

Kolhapur district of Maharashtra is one of the richest districts in India in terms of per capita income. It is well known for the temple of the goddess Mahalakshmi. Despite this background, as per the 2001 census, the sex ratio in Kolhapur was 839 girls per 1,000 boys. District Magistrate and Collector Laxmikant Deshmukh initiated the Save the Baby Girl drive, while Magnum Opus invented the instruments and implemented the project. The pilot was launched on 15 August 2009. Kolhapur district has 252 registered genetics centres, 120 in urban locations and 132 in rural areas. There are 280 USG machines across the district.

The innovation began by asking the following questions:

1. How can the number of pregnant females in the district be estimated?
2. How is it possible to find out who has had a sonography done, and at which centre?

3. How is it possible to find out which doctor performed the sonography?
4. How can one access the details regarding the pregnancy of the woman revealed through the sonography?

Save the Baby Girl and Active Tracker, a local initiative and a technological innovation, answered all these questions. Every sonography video is now recorded on the Active Tracker device, and online submissions of form F have increased from 8,000 forms per month to 16,000 forms per month.

The new system was challenged by the Indian Radiological and Imaging Association through a writ petition in the Bombay High Court, primarily on the grounds of concerns about patient privacy and the legality of the system. The Bombay High Court issued a historic judgement, stating that the right to life is more important than the right to privacy.[2] Thus, the invention obtained legal status. In May 2012, the Rajasthan High Court through its judgement made online submission of form F and the installation of Active Tracker mandatory for all registered sonography machines across the state of Rajasthan. The project had now been successfully implemented in Gwalior, Indore, and a few other districts of Madhya Pradesh, Punjab and Haryana.

The project offers an adequate solution to the problem of the declining female sex ratio as a result of the misuse of diagnostic technologies. Its merits have been recognised by various institutions and dignitaries. The project has also won various national awards, such as the National Association of Software and Services Companies Function Award, the eIndia Award, the Manthan Award, Maharashtra Foundation Award, Times of India Social Impact Award, Excellence in E-Governance Award of Madhya Pradesh, and so on. The project has been appreciated by various eminent individuals such as former president of India A. P. J. Abdul Kalam, Narayana Murthy, Nandan Nilekani, and many others. The programme has already been scaled up to the state level, and has the potential to be scaled to the national level.

Conclusion

Sex selection, and subsequent female foeticide, is a serious issue in India. It is not restricted to the illiterate, but cuts across all classes of literacy, economic and social status, and religion across India. Female discrimination is seen all over the world in varying degrees. Educating people through awareness campaigns is one way of reducing such discrimination, but it will take years to change the mindsets of millions of people. In the meantime, effective implementation of the PCPNDT Act would definitely allow thousands of baby girls to live.

The rationale for the project outlined in this chapter goes much beyond technology, foreseeing the disastrous future implications of the declining female sex ratio. Save the Baby Girl is an attempt to introduce technology to help administrators effectively implement the PCPNDT Act. Active Tracker is intended as a deterrent for doctors involved in the illegal practice of sex determination.

The ultimate purpose of the project is to save baby girls. Its success in Kolhapur district gives reasons for hope. The sex ratio in the district has increased from 839 girls per 1,000 boys as per the 2001 census, to 903 girls per 1,000 boys by March 2014. We sincerely appreciate the positive contribution of the doctors of Kolhapur and the Radiologist Association of Kolhapur for their unconditional support to this cause. Without them, the project would not have been successful.

—

Notes

1. Save the Baby Girl Initiative by District Administration, Kolhapur, www. savethebabygirl.org (accessed on 24 December 2014).
2. Bombay High Court, *Radiological and Imaging Association vs Union of India*, Writ Petition no. 797 of 2011, 26 August 2011, http://indiankanoon.org/doc/680703/ (accessed on 15 February 2011).

Reference

UNFPA (United Nations Population Fund), India. 2010. 'Trends in Sex Ratio at Birth and Estimates of Girls Missing at Birth in India', July, http://countryoffice.unfpa.org/india/drive/SRBBooklet.pdf (accessed on 24 December 2014).

2

Communication Trends among Hospital Personnel

A Multi-site Methodology

Candice D. Presseau, Qian Gao, Osman R. Sayan,
Elise Kang and Stan Kachnowski

■

Research on the use of technology made to address communication tendencies of healthcare professionals (HCPs) in hospitals has focused on small, homogeneous samples.[1] The objective of this chapter is to identify communication patterns of hospital personnel in various-sized hospitals from a diverse sample of HCPs. Healthcare personnel from four different hospitals were observed for 1–3 hours, and 3,200 communication events and attributes were recorded and codified. The conclusion reached was that synchronous communication was predominant. Events were characterised by interruptions (37.7 per cent), multi-tasking (14.2 per cent), and break-in-tasks (1.1 per cent). Communication trends among HCPs were similar across hospitals. Health information technology, despite its continued growth, was seldom used for communication purposes.

Background

Information management, including the transfer of information, is a critical component of healthcare. Accurate and timely management of patient information, enabled by effective communication strategies, leads to more efficient patient care. These components of care are particularly important in critical care settings such as hospitals, where the time-sensitivity of illnesses is heightened and timely access to complete and accurate information can be problematic. Moreover, in hospital settings, the skill of multi-tasking is essential since HCPs are often required to simultaneously care for multiple patients (Laxmisan et al. 2007). Healthcare professionals must care for many patients at once, all with differing levels of illness severity, and at different stages of evaluation and stabilisation. Interactions among hospital personnel, including resident physicians, medical students, nurses, pharmacists, clerks and technicians, become exceedingly necessary to ensure proper, error-free care. In hospital settings, interruptions often function as essential communication tools, alerting hospital personnel about urgent or potentially dangerous situations (Alvarez and Coiera 2005), and at times permitting important exchanges of information. It is clear from their well-established prevalence (Brixey, Robinson et al. 2010; Fairbanks et al. 2007) that interruptions serve a positive and preventative function (Grundgeiger and Sanderson 2009) that cannot be disregarded. Interruptions, however, can be a double-edged sword. Interruptions are by definition disruptive; they can impair workflow efficiency if they are not successfully used and/or triaged. Breakdowns in communication, common in highly interruptive environments like hospitals (Alvarez and Coiera 2005; Brixey, Tang et al. 2008; Coiera and Tombs 1998; Woloshynowych et al. 2007), lead to an increased likelihood of adverse events due to medical errors (Greenberg et al. 2007; Horwitz et al. 2009). It is for these reasons that much attention has been given to the issue of patient information transfer, as well as attempts to characterise and improve it.

To date, much of the work on communication within hospitals has strictly emphasised the physician–nurse communication and has excluded other integral HCPs. Communication trends have been found to vary among different categories of HCPs and even within different units of the same emergency department (Brixey, Robinson et al. 2010; Fairbanks et al. 2007; Laxmisan et al. 2007). Considering the interdependence of nurses, physicians, aides/technicians, pharmacists and all healthcare providers in the highly contained, interruptive hospital workspace, understanding communicative processes as they play out in real time is unequivocally valuable. This understanding can serve to guide the improvement of existing infrastructures. Therefore, research that furthers our understanding of the communication patterns among hospital personnel, including integral members such as pharmacists and lab technicians, is needed.

Efforts to fortify information management in healthcare have relied heavily on the use of technology — both hardware and information technology (IT). The pervasion of these technologies, particularly mobile technologies, into the market has intensified the need to study their use by initiators and recipients of interruptions (Brixey, Robinson et al. 2010), and the extent to which they have been integrated into communication patterns of different types of HCPs. Information technology has the potential to enhance interdepartmental hospital operations through more accessible documentation of communication and facilitation of interdisciplinary collaboration, which has been linked to acute care provider satisfaction (Dykes et al. 2006). In contrast, the failure to implement or integrate IT successfully into the workflow can lead to task duplication and to less efficient use of time and cognitive resources among hospital employees (Horsky et al. 2006). The relationship of IT to patient outcomes has already emerged as a rich area of intrigue (Fairbanks et al. 2007); however, attempts to elucidate technology utilisation for communication purposes have, thus far, been made only with respect to intra-hospital processes — organisation, information flow and staff workflow (Reddy et al. 2005; Zwarenstein et al. 2007).

Many of today's technologies have been designed mostly to address concerns about hospital-wide communication, yet qualitative investigations of communication tendencies in acute healthcare settings, serving as the basis for technological innovation, typically involve only one or two study sites and small samples of HCPs (Brixey, Tang et al. 2008; Coiera and Tombs 1998; Fairbanks et al. 2007; Spencer et al. 2004). Previous research indicates a prevalent bias on the part of HCPs towards synchronous, face-to-face methods of information exchange (Brixey, Tang et al. 2008; Fairbanks et al. 2007; Spencer et al. 2004; Woloshynowych et al. 2007), although these findings have not been confirmed using a multi-site methodology or with a diverse sample of HCPs. This study responded to the knowledge gap in this area using observations of multiple types of hospital professionals from a number of hospital sites in order to answer three specific questions: (a) how often are multi-tasking and interruption involved in the communication events of various hospital personnel; (b) what methods of information exchange are readily employed by HCPs in the hospital setting; and (c) how do findings differ across categories of HCPs in small, medium and large hospitals.

Methods

This qualitative, multi-site, observational study was carried out in four hospitals of various sizes throughout New York State with 800, 758, 627 and 235 beds, respectively. The hospitals containing more than 700 beds were classified as 'large' and the hospitals containing 627 and 235 beds were considered to be 'medium' and 'small' in size. A convenience sample of hospital employees belonging to the following job categories was selected for participation: physician (attending and resident), nurse, physician assistant (PA), laboratory technician and pharmacist. After receiving informed consent from HCPs at the study sites, researchers proceeded to shadow them unobtrusively for durations of 1–3 hours, a timeframe similar to that used in other studies (Coiera and Tombs 1998; Spencer et al. 2004), closely observing and documenting their behaviours. The shadowing method, reminiscent of the communication observation method employed by Spencer et al. (2004), has been used in other studies as a means of observing participants' performance of tasks in a real-world setting (Brixey, Tang et al. 2008). The method used herein involved the matching of one research assistant (RA) and one healthcare professional.

Outcome Measures

Patterns of communication were determined by classifying and documenting attributes of communication events, including: clinician being observed, channels of communication relied upon, purpose of the event, event duration, agents/initiators of interruptions, recipients of interruptions, use of multi-tasking, and break-in-tasks associated with the event. 'Observation events' were considered to be the 1–3 hour intervals during which participants were shadowed. A 'communication event' was defined as any action taken in order to relay information to another clinician, including conversations, telephone calls, faxes, pages, emails, voicemails, notes written in a patient record and text messages. Delay or lack of information retrieval by the intended recipient was not a criterion for classification as a communication event. An 'interruption' was defined as any disruptive activity, clinician conversation, event or alert that occurred during a communication stream between two healthcare providers. 'Multi-tasking' was defined as attending to more than one duty at the same time while attempting to communicate (i.e., during a communication event) with another clinician. A 'break-in-task' was considered to be the extinction of a duty or task that was not resumed during a communication event, although the task could be resumed at some point during the observation event.

Any disruptions in communication flows were also noted during observation events, as well as behaviours that sought to compensate for inefficient communication. Qualitative observations were limited to the aforementioned methodology and included no structured interviews between RAs and participants. Verbal interactions between RAs and participants were also kept to a minimum, except for instances in which clarification on observations was needed. The RAs did not collect or document information on participant demographics. Permission was obtained from the Institutional Review Board (IRB) at each hospital before RAs were permitted entrance. All researchers were certified with the necessary Health Insurance Portability and Accountability Act (HIPAA) and Good Clinical Practice requirements. The security, confidentiality and protection of participants' data were maintained.

Data Collection and Analysis

Research assistants observed and documented their observations using a pre-established coding scheme. The RAs were trained with regard to the system and method of coding to ensure consistency among RAs. The RAs documented all communication events that occurred during the observation timeframe in addition to all tasks completed and/or attempted on a field worksheet, and tracked time using hand-held, synchronised digital stopwatches. The field worksheet was a paper-based, semi-structured observation tool. The data were coded in a manner conducive to tabulation by research analysts, both during and following observation periods, and entered into a study-specific Microsoft® Access database for analysis that conformed to IRB and HIPAA standards.

Data from each hospital were exported to SPSS® for Windows (Version 14.0) and then merged into a single data set containing information from all study sites. Descriptive statistics (i.e., frequency and percentages) were used to characterise communication patterns of hospital personnel (interruptions, multi-tasking and break-in-tasks) and the employment of communication methods, within and across study sites.

Results

A total of 3,200 communication events were observed, comprising 85.3 per cent (5,485.0 minutes) of the total observation time (6,431.3 minutes) over 55 observation events (sd = 53.0 minutes) as shown in Table 2.1. Of these, 2,107 communication events were observed in the two large hospitals, 862 in the medium-sized hospital, and 231 in the small hospital. Of these observations, the majority (85.3 per cent) occurred within an emergency department (i.e., general, fast-track, paediatric, or prompt care emergency department), with 200 taking place in a hospital pharmacy (6.3 per cent), 76 (2.4 per cent) in a critical care trauma unit, 57 (1.8 per cent) in a radiology department, 53 (1.7 per cent) on an internal medicine floor, 45 (1.4 per cent) in a lab-central processing centre, and 38 (1.2 per cent) in an intensive care unit (ICU). Communication events among attending physicians comprised 52 per cent (n = 1,681) of the total events observed, whereas

Table 2.1 Frequency of Communication
Events by Subject of Observation

Subject of Observation	Communication Events n (%), Total N = 3,200
Hospital size	
Large	2,107 (65.8)
Medium	862 (26.9)
Small	231 (7.2)
Department	
Emergency (general, fast-track, paediatrics, prompt care)	2,731 (85.3)
Pharmacy	200 (6.3)
Critical care trauma	76 (2.4)
Radiology	57 (1.8)
Internal medicine floor	53 (1.7)
Lab-central processing	45 (1.4)
ICU	38 (1.2)
Hospital personnel	
Attending physician	1,681 (52.5)
Nurse	818 (25.6)
Resident	422 (13.2)
Pharmacist	200 (6.3)
Lab technician	47 (1.5)
PA	32 (1.0)

Source: Based on the authors' observations during the research.

nurse (n = 818; 25.6 per cent), resident physician (n = 422; 13.2 per cent), pharmacist (n = 200; 6.3 per cent), lab technician (n = 47; 1.5 per cent), and PA (n = 32; 1.0 per cent) participants were involved in the remaining 48 per cent of communication event observations.

Hospital personnel, with the exception of lab technicians and pharmacists, were more likely to be the initiators (n = 1,964; 61.4 per cent) of communication than to be receivers (n = 1,236; 38.6 per cent), and the same was found for large (61.1 per cent), medium (58.7 per cent) and small (74.0 per cent) hospitals. Communication events involved interruption 37.7 per cent of the time, with 43.4 per cent of interruptions initiated by the professional being shadowed. Although hospital professionals more frequently initiated communication events, they rarely initiated communication events that involved interruptions. Pharmacists were the only professionals shadowed whose communication events involved a majority, but only a slight majority, of interruptions (54.0 per cent). Physician assistants were found to more often initiate than receive interruptions (i.e., 66.7 per cent of interruptions were initiated by PAs), although there was a relatively low number of communication events involving interruptions (n = 12) observed compared to those for other clinician categories, such as nurses (n = 352) and attending physicians (n = 612).

Resident physicians, on the other hand, were interrupted during communication events less than any other hospital professional types (23.9 per cent). Resident physicians were also found to be recipients of interruptions (77.2 per cent) more often than initiators compared to other job categories, despite their lower incidence of interruptions. Attending physicians shadowed were predominantly recipients, as opposed to initiators, of interruptions at high frequencies as well. Nurses and physicians were more often recipients than initiators of interruptions. Nurses (47.4 per cent) initiated interruptions more often than physicians, although attending physicians (44.6 per cent) initiated interruptions only slightly less than nurses while resident physicians (22.8 per cent) initiated interruptions much less than nurses.

Multi-tasking was involved in communication events 14.2 per cent of the time with comparable findings for all job categories. Pharmacists were involved in communication events that led to the most multi-tasking (26.0 per cent) and nurses, the least (9.6 per cent). Break-in-tasks associated with communication events were extremely uncommon, occurring for 1.1 per cent (n = 36) of the communication events and again yielding similar percentages for all job categories (range 0.0 per cent to 2.6 per cent). Comparable results regarding the incidence of communication event types were also obtained for small-, medium- and large-sized hospitals. Hospitals had progressively fewer interruptions as size decreased with 40.5 per cent, 35.7 per cent and 19.0 per cent of communications involving interruptions at large, medium and small hospitals, respectively.

Face-to-face contact was the most common method of information exchange used during communication events overall (69.8 per cent) and for all job categories (Table 2.2). The communication events of nurses (79.7 per cent), PAs (68.8 per cent) and attending physicians (67.4 per cent) more frequently relied on face-to-face contact as compared to other categories of hospital personnel, such as lab technicians (46.8 per cent) and pharmacists (63.5 per cent). Landline phones (12.4 per cent), hospital computerised systems (9.7 per cent), paper/medical charts (5.9 per cent) and paper forms (3.5 per cent) were the other commonly used forms of communication. The pharmacist category yielded the highest frequency (1.5 per cent) of

Table 2.2 Frequency of Communication Methods Employed during Communication Events

Method of Communication	Communication Events n (%), Total N = 3,200
Face-to-face	2,234 (69.8)
Landline phone	398 (12.4)
Hospital computerised system	309 (9.7)
Paper chart/medical record	188 (5.9)
Paper form	111 (3.5)
Electronic medical record	90 (2.8)
Cell phone/mobile phone	70 (2.2)
Written note on paper	61 (1.9)
Overhead pager/PA system	44 (1.4)
Beeper/pager	31 (1.0)
PDA/smartphone	19 (0.6)
Log book	16 (0.5)
Fax	7 (0.2)
Email	4 (0.1)
Text message	3 (0.1)
Electronic white board	3 (0.1)
Notice board	3 (0.1)
Voicemail	2 (0.1)

Source: Based on data collected during the research.

fax usage for communication purposes, while fax (0.2 per cent), text message (0.1 per cent), email (0.1 per cent), electronic whiteboard (0.1 per cent), notice board (0.1 per cent) and voicemail (0.1 per cent) were the least frequently employed methods of communicating information among all hospital personnel job categories.

Attending physicians, resident physicians and nurses more readily employed multiple modes of communication as compared to other job categories, using electronic medical records (EMRs), personal digital assistants (PDAs) or smartphones, written notes on paper, cell/mobile phones and beepers/pagers as means of communication at greater frequencies than other categories. The results suggest that these categories of professionals are most technologically inclined, or rather, that these mediums are more accessible by these categories of hospital personnel. Those categorised as lab technicians (14.9 per cent) and PAs (6.3 per cent) were most likely to participate in communication events involving paper forms, whereas PA and pharmacist job categorisations most frequently used landline phones during communication events (28.1 per cent and 24.0 per cent, respectively).

Both similarities and differences in the frequency of use for different methods of communication were also observed with respect to hospital size. Interestingly, EMRs were used to communicate information less frequently as hospital size increased, although hospital personnel tended to use hand-written notes more often as hospital size decreased. The small hospital study site was the least likely to use a hospital computerised system (4.3 per cent) during communication events when compared to medium (13.9 per cent) and large (8.5 per cent) hospitals. These findings imply that hospitals, regardless of size, rely on multiple methods for information exchange; however, they support the contention that hospitals of different sizes do vary in the communication methods they employ. Taken together, hospitals were found to use cellular and mobile phones, PDAs/smartphones, faxes, and beepers/pagers during less than 5.0 per cent of their communication events.

Comment

Although some variations in the characteristics of communication events were observed, hospital personnel within and across hospitals were quite similar in their communication practices, as they typically relied on synchronous channels of communication and were involved in communication events they had initiated. In addition, communication events involved interruptions that were more often initiated by others and rarely led to break-in-tasks. These findings suggest that even though hospital personnel are persistently met with communication demands, they are generally successful at completing the tasks they are involved in, either preceding or following the communication event.

The study findings provide evidence both in support of and contrary to existing findings, further illuminating the importance of repeated examinations of these issues. Brixey, Tang et al. (2008) surmise that their observance of greater frequencies of interruption events for nurses compared to physicians was related to the multi-tasking nature of nursing which requires nurses to attend readily to a variety of responsibilities and duties. In contrast, our findings show that nurses and physicians are involved in communication events that have nearly equivalent proportions of both interruptions and multi-tasking. In fact, hospital personnel participated in communication events involving interruptions and multi-tasking at similar frequencies. Nurses were, in contrast to Brixey's finding, engaged in communication events involving the least amount of multi-tasking. This study's finding that communication events among pharmacists involved the highest frequency of multi-tasking and more interruptions than nurses is one that warrants further examination, as this result has not been reported previously. Interestingly, none of the 200 communication events observed for pharmacists led to break-in-tasks. Pharmacists, although largely unexamined in previous observations, are particularly effective at navigating the communication processes in which they are involved but do not tend to initiate. The same trend can be noted, though less distinctively, in the communication patterns of all job categories supporting previous findings that clinicians are able to continue performing the tasks to which they were attending before being interrupted (Laxmisan et al. 2007). It is important to keep in mind that these findings are only indicative of participants' involvement in multi-tasking during communication events and do not suggest that particular categories of HCP were, or are, more or less involved in multi-tasking during the whole of the observation event or thereafter.

Our study's size and scale are instrumental in iterating the consistency and inconsistency of communication patterns within and across different hospitals, thereby substantiating intuitive suppositions about the ways that HCPs interact with one another in addition to those reported in smaller-scale studies. For example, our data support the finding that nurses and physicians are more likely to receive rather than initiate interruptions and that nurses are more likely to be initiators of interruptions than physicians (Brixey, Tang et al. 2008). Previously, attending physicians, compared to resident physicians, were reported to engage in interruptions and multi-tasking at higher frequencies (Laxmisan et al. 2007) and differential interruption rates have been reported for the same types of personnel in different arms (i.e., adult and paediatric) of the same emergency department (Fairbanks et al. 2007). Our data indicate that attending physicians are involved in interruptions more frequently than residents but multi-task less and have fewer break-in-tasks. These discrepancies in communication tendencies among HCPs within and across hospitals must be acknowledged, as the detection of these differences reminds us that there is no universal approach to information exchange, delivery of care or inter-clinician communication within or across hospitals.

Our study synthesised observations of a variety of hospital providers using a multi-site methodology, thereby achieving a total observation time that exceeds those of previous studies. Other studies using similar methodology to examine communication among hospital personnel have involved one or two study sites and small, homogeneous samples of healthcare providers (Brixey, Tang et al. 2008; Fairbanks et al. 2007; Horsky et al. 2006; Spencer et al. 2004; Woloshynowych et al. 2007). A number of these studies have observed participants for periods of approximately 20 to 40 hours (Fairbanks et al. 2007; Spencer et al. 2004; Woloshynowych et al. 2007), nearly 60 hours less than our study. One study included as few as 831 communication events (Spencer et al. 2004), while another observed 1,665 communication events, which is also much lower than our observation of 3,200 communication events. The results of our study highlight the importance and relevance of qualitative investigations, as they provide detailed observations of the communication tools and practices employed by healthcare providers.

Although many of the limitations of the existing literature are related to the nature of the qualitative approach, a larger sample and increased number of observations have served to meaningfully elucidate communication practices among HCPs. At the same time, however, the use of a larger sample required that several RAs conduct the observations, potentially leading to differences in coding and the classifying of events. No measures of inter-rater reliability were obtained. Thus, the consistency of observer coding among observers is unknown. Moreover, the inability of researchers to interact with participants during the observation period may have caused some uncertainty about participants' behaviours. Even though RAs were encouraged to gain clarification in these instances, it is still unknown to what extent clarification was achieved and subsequently indicated in the data gathered. It is likely that issues of uncharted ambiguity emerged during data collection. Additionally, time and day of observation were not consistent for all categories of hospital personnel or for all of the four hospitals, which could have introduced another source of variability into the results.

A final limitation emerges with respect to interpretability of findings, as RAs did not indicate during the observation events which methods of communication were available to hospital personnel. It remains largely unknown whether the findings obtained indicate differences in utilisation of communication methods that result from the hospital's size alone or are due to other intermediary factors (e.g., access to technology, training, cost or participant preference) that may have determined participants' selection of communication approach. For example, frequencies of use for different methods of communication may have been influenced by the availability, or lack thereof, of mediums of information transfer as well as their integration into the hospital workflow. Unfortunately, this line of reasoning is not supported by the data collected during, prior to, or following observation events.

Despite the study's limitations, many of which are common to qualitative research investigations, identification of communication patterns as they surface in multiple hospital sites and for a variety of HCPs is useful for designing interventions that meet the needs of different categories of hospital healthcare providers. Strategies for the design and integration of technologies operate under the assumption that something is flawed in communications as they occur at present; however, the evidence obtained through this investigation suggests that hospital personnel are aptly responsive to their tasks during communication events despite the limited use of asynchronous methods of communicating. Considering the plethora of communication devices and modes of information exchange available to hospitals alongside their limited usage, it is unclear whether providers have been given sufficient access to these communication resources and if integration of newly developed systems has taken place within hospitals. If the purpose of IT application and implementation as a means of enhancing communication capabilities and interdisciplinary information exchange has not been adequately conveyed to care providers, their functionality may remain questionable and their usability low. It is conceivable that improving communicativeness among healthcare providers should focus on reducing the time required for communication events and reducing HCPs' need for direct face-to-face communication by making information more accessible and transmittance of information occur more swiftly. The availability and use of EMRs as opposed to paper charts, for example, has already been demonstrated as a means through which documentation can be improved (Wu and Straus 2006). The disproportionate use of EMRs observed across categories of HCPs and hospitals of different sizes in this study suggests that integration of EMRs into hospital workflow and communication interchange would introduce increased capabilities of such a magnitude that would lead to more productive, efficient, and less interruptive communication practices. Providing members of the healthcare community as well as patients themselves access to EMRs could alter the landscape of information retrieval and delivery both in and outside of the hospital by extending the reach of IT initiatives beyond the scope of communication triage. Such information exchanges could impact the internal operations and communication processes not only within hospitals but also at the systems level by reducing communication load and providing a less error-prone, comprehensive flow of patient information (Laxmisan et al. 2007).

Changes imposed on the system of healthcare should, on the other hand, be made only to the extent that they can adapt and respond to the differing components of that system and modulate the enduring inefficiencies found within it. Even though IT strategies for facilitating communication have been associated with greater satisfaction by nurses and other acute care providers (Dykes et al. 2006) and have led to reductions in interruptive information transfers in nurse–physician interactions (Laxmisan et al. 2007), future investigations must further examine the extent to which the unavailability of IT, both in terms of physical presence in the workplace and lack of integration into the workflow, serves to hinder its use by hospital personnel and/or HCPs.

—

Note

1. This project was supported by a grant received from Qualcomm® Enterprise Services. Qualcomm® did not participate in the design or conduct of the study, nor was the organisation involved in the collection, management, analysis and interpretation of data or the preparation, review and approval of the manuscript for publication. We greatly appreciate Qualcomm's willingness to fund our initiative while allowing us the freedom to conduct, complete and publish our findings independently. We would also like to extend our thanks to the study participants who willingly volunteered to be observed and to take part in the study. We appreciate also the administrators at all of the four hospitals who permitted us to conduct the study in their facilities and to use their space and resources for the length of the study. Contributions: Candice Presseau wrote and revised several drafts of the manuscript and was assisted primarily by Qian Gao, who also completed the statistical analyses and created tables and figures as needed. Qian Gao had full access to all the data in the study and takes responsibility for the integrity of the data and the accuracy of the data analysis. Dr Osman Sayan made significant revisions to intellectual content of the manuscript during the editing phase, playing a critical role in preparing the manuscript for submission. Stan Kachnowski played a key managing role in the execution of the study and throughout the conception and writing of the manuscript, providing direction and expertise that were extremely helpful. Sara Augustine was heavily involved in the study design and conduct, and helped create a framework in which the study findings could be considered using relevant research findings. Ilene Hollin contributed to the preparation of this manuscript. A special thank you also to our HIT Lab team and alumni including: Ashley Edwards, Leslie-Anne Fitzpatrick, Angie Cheng and Alex Trzebucki, who were heavily involved in the study's design, conduct, data collection and preliminary data analyses.

References

Alvarez, G., and E. Coiera (2005). 'Interruptive Communication Patterns in the Intensive Care Unit Ward Round', *International Journal of Medical Informatics*, vol. 74, no. 10, pp. 791–96.

Brixey, J. J., D. J. Robinson, J. P. Turley and J. Zhang (2010). 'The Roles of MDs and RNs as Initiators and Recipients of Interruptions in Workflow', *International Journal of Medical Informatics*, vol. 79, no. 6, pp. e109–15.

Brixey, J. J., Z. Tang, D. J. Robinson, C. W. Johnson, T. R. Johnson, J. P. Turley, V. L. Patel and J. Zhang (2008). 'Interruptions in a Level One Trauma Center: A Case Study', *International Journal of Medical Informatics*, vol. 77, no. 4, pp. 235–41.

Coiera, E., and V. Tombs (1998). 'Communication Behaviours in a Hospital Setting: An Observational Study', *BMJ*, vol. 316, no. 7132, pp. 673–76.

Dykes, P., M. Cashen, M. Foster, J. Gallagher, M. Kennedy, R. Maccalum, J. Murphy, R. Schleyer and S. Whetstone (2006). 'Surveying Acute Care Providers in the US to Explore the Impact of Health Information Technology on the Role of Nurses and Interdisciplinary Communication in Acute Care Settings', *Computers Informatics Nursing*, vol. 24, no. 6, pp. 353–54.

Fairbanks, R. J., A. M. Bisantz and M. Sunm (2007). 'Emergency Department Communication Links and Patterns', *Annals of Emergency Medicine*, vol. 50, no. 5, pp. 396–406.

Greenberg, C. C., S. E. Regenbogen, D. M. Studdert, S. R. Lipsitz, S. O. Rogers, M. J. Zinner and A. A. Gawande (2007). 'Patterns of Communication Breakdowns Resulting in Injury to Surgical Patients', *Journal of the American College of Surgeons*, vol. 204, no. 4, pp. 533–40.

Grundgeiger, T., and P. Sanderson (2009). 'Interruptions in Healthcare: Theoretical Views', *International Journal of Medical Informatics*, vol. 78, no. 5, pp. 293–307.

Horsky, J., L. Gutnik and V. L. Patel (2006). 'Technology for Emergency Care: Cognitive and Workflow Considerations', *AMIA Annual Symposium Proceedings*, vol. 2006, pp. 344–448.

Horwitz, L. I., T. Meredith, J. D. Schuur, N. R. Shah, R. G. Kulkarni and G. Y. Jeng (2009). 'Dropping the Baton: A Qualitative Analysis of Failures during the Transition from Emergency Department to Inpatient Care', *Annals of Emergency Medicine*, vol. 53, no. 6, pp. 701–10.e4.

Laxmisan, A., F. Hakimzadaa, O. R. Sayan, R. A. Green and V. L. Patel (2007). 'The Multitasking Clinician: Decision-Making and Cognitive Demand During and After Team Handoffs in Emergency Care', *International Journal of Medical Informatics*, vol. 76, pp. 801–11.

Reddy, M. C., D. W. McDonald, W. Pratt and M. M. Shabot (2005). 'Technology, Work, and Information Flows: Lessons from the Implementation of a Wireless Alert Pager System', *Journal of Biomedical Informatics*, vol. 38, no. 3, pp. 229–38.

Spencer, R., E. Coiera and P. Logan (2004). 'Variation in Communication Loads on Clinical Staff in the Emergency Department', *Annals of Emergency Medicine*, vol. 44, no. 3, pp. 268–73.

Woloshynowych, M., R. Davis, R. Brown and C. Vincent (2007). 'Communication Patterns in a UK Emergency Department', *Annals of Emergency Medicine*, vol. 50, no. 4, pp. 407–13.

Wu, R. C., and S. E. Straus (2006). 'Evidence for Handheld Electronic Medical Records in Improving Care: A Systematic Review', *BMC Medical Informatics and Decision Making*, vol. 6, p. 26.

Zwarenstein, M., S. Reeves, A. Russell, C. Kenaszchuk, L. G. Conn, L. L. Miller, L. Lingard and K. E. Thorpe (2007). 'Structuring Communication Relationships for Interprofessional Teamwork (SCRIPT): A Cluster Randomised Controlled Trial', *Trials*, vol. 8, p. 23.

3

Measuring Service Quality in Health Sectors Using the SERVQUAL Model

Chhanda Ray and Manigrib Bag

◘

In recent years, the services sector has been growing very rapidly with the advancement of the economy, leading to greater employment opportunities. With intensifying competition in most service industries, it has become progressively more important for the services sector to provide quality services to consumers. Service quality is typically defined in terms of customer satisfaction. Customer satisfaction is the feeling or attitude of a customer towards a product or service after it has been used. A major outcome of customer satisfaction is a stream of profitable revenue resulting from their own patronage of a service as well as from others to whom they recommend the services used by them. Moreover, customer satisfaction is widely recognised as a key influence in the formation of customers' future purchase intentions. This scenario is also true for healthcare organisations.

In today's era, patients are very conscious about the quality of treatment and care processes provided by health sector organisations. In health sector organisations, patients are considered as customers, while physicians or the authorities of hospitals are perceived as the purveyors of services. In India, a patient has the opportunity to file a case against any physician or healthcare authority through a consumer forum if he/she does not feel satisfied with the treatment and care provided by a healthcare organisation. In recent times, the concept of patient satisfaction has been the focus of attention for many healthcare organisations in the light of the fact that patients are the primary sources of most organisations' revenue. However, a consensual definition of the concept has not yet emerged.

Literature Survey

Patient satisfaction is the key to the success of healthcare organisations, and this has led the healthcare sector to improve its service quality and care processes continuously in order to maximise patient satisfaction. In 1992, the Patients' Bill of Rights was adopted by the American Hospital Association (AHA Board of Trustees 1992). Strassar and Scheweikhart (1994) show that different healthcare organisations demonstrate the importance of patient satisfaction as a measure of health service quality. Maryland Mental Health Partners published a report on Consumer Satisfaction and Outcomes in 1999 (Oliver et al. 1999) in which they achieved 77.9 per cent responses in favour of patient satisfaction. In July 1997, the Public Mental Health System of Maryland was launched (ibid.) along with special services of interviews with consumers to assess satisfaction. Croze (1994) states that treatment should be limited by consumers, which will help to control access and thereby control costs. From the studies cited so far, it may be inferred that healthcare purchases must be responsive to consumers and their family members, and the means of ensuring this are to be developed by their meaningful participation in treatment decisions, measurement of satisfaction and measurement of treatment effectiveness.

Due to unequal socio-economic status and the complex nature of human beings, achieving customer satisfaction is a very trivial task. Customer satisfaction is generally described as the full meeting of one's expectations (Oliver and Swan 1989). Satisfaction and service quality are often treated as functions of a customer's perceptions and expectations (Swartz and Brown 1989). Service quality is reported to have apparent relationships to costs, profitability, customer satisfaction, customer retention, behavioural intention and positive word of mouth. Parasuraman et al. (1985) developed a conceptual model for service quality. Later, the same authors (Parasuraman et al. 1988) described service quality as the ability of an organisation to meet or exceed customer expectations. In recent years, greater emphasis has been placed on the need to understand the role of expectations, given the fact that consumers' expectations of quality are increasing, and people are becoming more discerning and critical of the quality of service that they experience. Oliver and Swan (1989) argue that the comparison between perception and expectation is the measure of customer satisfaction. If the perceived performance of any product or service exceeds the expectation of customers and consumers, then they will be satisfied. But if there is any shortfall between the perceived performance of any product or service and the expectation, the customer will be dissatisfied. Swartz and Brown (1989) draw some distinctions between different views on service quality based on the works of Gronroos (1988) and Lehtinen and Lehtinen (1982) concerning the dimensions of service quality.

Further empirical scrutiny has been conducted on a 22-item scale, called 'SERVQUAL', which measures service quality based on the dimensions of tangibles, reliability, responsiveness, assurance and empathy (Parasuraman et al. 1988). Empirical assessments of the SERVQUAL scale are provided in Babakus and Boller (1992), and Brown and Swartz (1989). Carman (1990) offers an assessment of the SERVQUAL dimensions for consumer perceptions of service quality. Richard and Allaway (1993) focus on service quality attributes and choice behaviour, while the gap in professional service quality has been analysed in Brown and Swartz (1989).

The objective of this chapter is to measure the service quality of healthcare units in India in the light of the comprehensive SERVQUAL model. The organisation of this chapter is as follows. The healthcare facility and customer satisfaction are discussed in the next section. Details of service quality models are introduced next. The chapter then represents service quality measurement in health sector organisations, before making some concluding observations.

The Healthcare Facility and Customer Satisfaction

Customer satisfaction is a customer-driven concept which allows customers to be in control of the system. Customer satisfaction is the collective outcome of the customer's perception, evaluation and psychological reaction with regard to the consumption experience of a product or a service. As customer satisfaction is commonly acknowledged as one of the most useful measurements of system success, organisations must identify the underlying factors of customer satisfaction and develop an instrument to measure these factors in order to be successful. Since the literature does not provide a unique conceptualisation of customer satisfaction, satisfaction can be considered as the consumer's fulfilment response. Most companies track customer satisfaction using a five-point scale: very dissatisfied, somewhat dissatisfied, indifferent, satisfied and very satisfied. In this context, the level of satisfaction is measured not only on an overall basis but also for each component of the company's offerings. Currently, the most widely adopted description of customer satisfaction is as a process, an evaluation of what was received and what was expected. Consequently, much research effort has been directed at understanding the cognitive processes involved in satisfaction evaluations. Equality theory has also been applied to customer satisfaction. According to this theory, individuals compare their input/output ratios with those of others. There are two principal interpretations of satisfaction within the literature — satisfaction as a process and satisfaction as an outcome. However, these are complementary interpretations, since often one depends on the other.

Like other business organisations, healthcare organisations have realised that treatment or service characteristics, the customer's aspirations and perceptions, and the availability of competitive alternatives can be used to enhance the value for money that consumers are looking for. In the global era, the main challenge of each healthcare organisation is to establish itself as an excellent service provider in order to achieve patient satisfaction. In India, people are no longer satisfied with average treatment or care processes, since they constantly experience high prices and thus expect superior quality services.

Unlike material products or pure services, most hospitality experiences are an amalgam of products and services. Therefore, satisfaction with a hospitality experience is a sum of total satisfactions with the individual elements or attributes of all services that make up the experience. There is no uniformity of opinion among marketing experts about the classification of elements in service encounters. Some researchers classify these elements into the functional element and the service, while others classify them as direct and indirect services. A more reasonable classification is in terms of essential attributes and subsidiary attributes. However, most researchers support the idea that service encounter attributes are situation-specific, and as such cannot be classified into universal elements.

In the context of healthcare organisations, service encounter attributes can be classified into two distinct categories: treatment attributes and other services attributes. Treatment attributes specify the quality of treatment provided by a particular healthcare organisation, and depend on the knowledge, efficiency and experience of physicians and staff, modernised medical equipment, the treatment facilities available, costs of treatment, etc. Similarly, other services attributes depend on the behaviour, caring and politeness of the staff, administration and physicians (in interactions with patients), infrastructure, cleanness, hygiene, food, timings, promptness of provision of services against any need, service delivery process, indirect services available, etc. (i.e., the overall environment of the healthcare organisation).

In the healthcare services, it is very important to note whether a change can improve the overall quality of treatment, the administration of healthcare organisations, and the infrastructure of hospitals. Even if a change can bring about an overall improvement in the health service, the question arises as to whether this improved and modernised service can fulfil the requirement of patients. In the Indian scenario, well-reputed private hospitals may provide quality services, but most people cannot afford the cost of treatment since such hospitals are quite expensive. On the other hand, government hospitals purvey the cheapest services to patients below the poverty line. These government hospitals can also provide good support during crises like rail and road accidents, natural calamities, etc. Therefore, achieving patient satisfaction in healthcare organisations in India is a very complicated task.

Patient satisfaction measurement serves two roles: providing information and enabling communication with patients. The primary reason for taking the time to measure patient satisfaction is to collect information, either regarding what patients say needs to be done differently, or to assess how well a healthcare unit is currently meeting its patients' needs. A secondary, but not less important, reason is that by surveying patients, a healthcare organisation is demonstrating its interest in communicating with its patients — finding out their needs, pleasures, displeasures and overall well-being.

Satisfaction and service quality are often treated together as functions of a customer's perceptions and expectations. Successful service quality strategies are generally characterised by customer segmentation, customer service, guarantees, continuous customer feedback and comprehensive measurement of organisation performance. The experience in many industries and organisations demonstrates that this process, although generally acknowledged, is not universally implemented. To measure service quality in healthcare organisations, some important points should be considered, such as:

- In services, every interaction between a patient and a service provider is a 'moment of truth'. Patient dis/satisfaction is a function of the difference between expected and perceived service. Hence, service quality is inherently defined in terms of patient dis/satisfaction.
- 'Patient complaints' are the broadest measure of quality available in healthcare organisations.
- The impact of factors such as holidays, natural calamities and some unavoidable situations can exhibit trends on quality and potentially introduce noise.

The purpose of resolving the issues just mentioned is to provide a better understanding of the satisfaction level of patients with regard to healthcare organisations, and of how such organisations can improve their service quality in order to maximise patient satisfaction.

Service Quality Models

In the literature, the construct of 'service quality' centres on perceived quality, defined as a consumer's judgement about an entity's overall excellence or superiority. Customer perceptions and expectations of service quality are increasingly used to forecast company profitability and prospects. To understand the main concepts under the umbrella of service quality, many conceptual quality models have been postulated. However, it would be impossible to ensure service quality in any organisation without determining the salient aspects of the service. In one attempt, seven service attributes have been listed that adequately embrace the concept of service quality, namely, security (confidence as well as physical safety), consistency (receiving the same quality of service each time), attitude (politeness and social manners), completeness (ancillary services available), condition (of facilities), availability (access, location and frequency) and training.

In other attempts (Gronroos 1988; Lehtinen and Lehtinen 1982), three dimensions of service quality have been suggested, namely, technical quality of the outcome, the functional quality of the encounter, and the company corporate image. A more recent conceptualisation proposes three dimensions of service quality as follows:

- the customer–employee interaction (that is, functional or process quality)
- the service environment, and
- the outcome (that is, technical quality).

The credit for pioneering service quality research goes to Parasuraman et al. (1988), a study whose service quality dimensions are most widely reported. According to Parasuraman et al. (ibid.), the criteria used by consumers that are important in moulding their expectations and perceptions of the delivered service fit into 10 dimensions, including tangibles, reliability, responsiveness, communications, credibility, security, competence, courtesy, understanding/knowing the customer and access. These are subsequently condensed into five dimensions of service performance known as SERVQUAL, namely, tangibles, reliability, responsiveness, assurance and empathy. The five SERVQUAL dimensions are a concise representation of the core criteria that customers employ in evaluating service quality. The SERVQUAL instrument was designed to measure service quality across a range of businesses such as retail banks, long-distance telephone companies, securities brokers, appliance repair and maintenance firms, and credit card companies.

Accepting the general validity of the SERVQUAL model, which assesses gaps between customer expectations of service quality and their perceptions of actual service delivery by the provider, the model has been adopted by international markets from earlier domestic applications. However, the SERVQUAL instrument focuses on functional quality dimensions and does not include any measure of the technical quality dimension. A more complete representation of service quality (Gronroos 1988; Lehtinen and Lehtinen 1982) includes three dimensions — technical, functional and image — as shown in Figure 3.1.

In this chapter, the comprehensive SERVQUAL model is adopted to measure service quality in health sector organisations. The measurement of service quality in healthcare organisations will help to

Figure 3.1 Gronroos's Service Quality Model

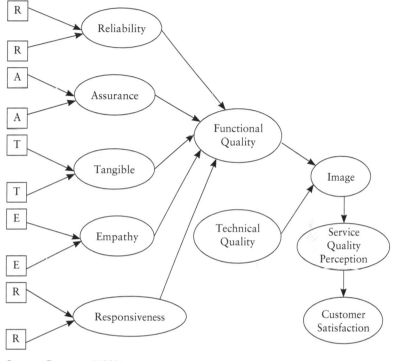

Source: Gronroos (1988).

judge patient satisfaction level. This will also help to determine how healthcare organisations can improve and enhance their treatment and services in order to achieve patient satisfaction.

Service Quality Measurement in Health Sectors

The service quality literature initially focused on measurement issues. In the SERVQUAL model, attention is centred on the determinants of perceived service quality, with particular emphasis on the service delivery process. A widely used method of measuring service quality in a generic service is the gap analysis model originally developed by Parasuraman et al. (1988). Our adaptation of the SERVQUAL model to measure service quality in the healthcare sector concentrates on five 'gaps' impairing the delivery of excellent service quality with a specific focus on gap 5, the difference between patient expectations and perceptions of service in the health sector. This modified SERVQUAL model is shown in Figure 3.2.

Figure 3.2 The SERVQUAL Model

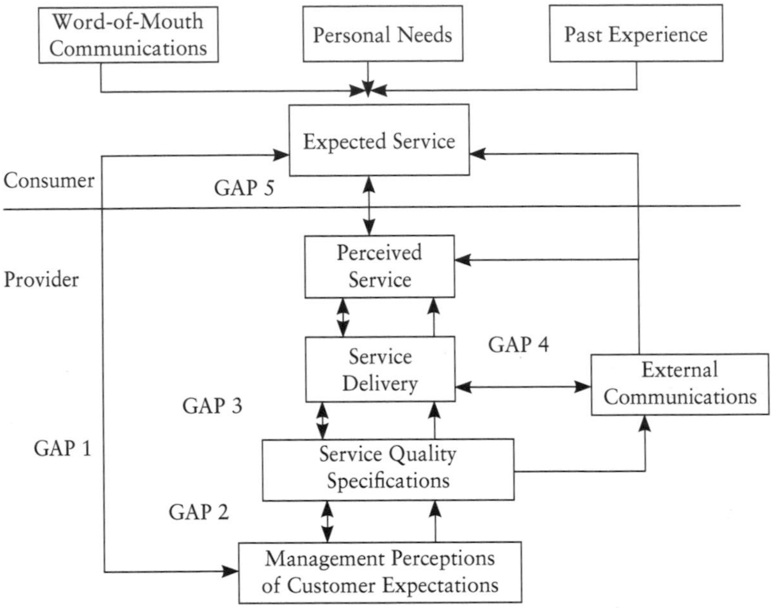

Source: Parasuraman et al. (1988).

In the context of the health sector in India, the details of measurement of service quality based on the seven service attributes — tangibles, reliability, responsiveness, assurance, empathy, technical and image — are presented in Table 3.1.

Conclusion and Future Work

The provision of high-quality, affordable healthcare services is an increasingly difficult challenge. This study focused on the service quality measurement of health sector organisations in India based on the comprehensive SERVQUAL model. The outcome of this measurement will provide a clear idea to healthcare organisations

Table 3.1 Service Dimensions and Measurement

TAN1	Availability of treatment for different diseases, different types of medical tests, and specialist physicians and staff
TAN2	Emergency treatment needs for patients and provision for 24-hour emergency medical services
TAN3	Cost of treatment and location of healthcare centres
TAN4	Appearance, attitudes and uniforms of physicians and staff
TAN5	Modern infrastructure, modern medical equipment, hygiene and cleanness of healthcare centres
TAN6	Availability of sufficient light and air and attached toilet in patient's room
TAN7	Variety and quality of food for patients
TAN8	Variety and choice of entertainment facilities
TAN9	Provision of video recording facilities during surgery and videos for healthcare facilities
REL1	Efficiency of patient's admission process
REL2	Efficiency of patient transfer process and discharge process
REL3	On-time performance in patient's treatment and care
REL4	Remedial procedures during holidays, natural calamities, etc.
REL5	Provision of all services regarding treatment and healthcare consistently
REL6	Performance of services right the first time
RES1	Capability of response and handling of emergency situations
RES2	Promptness of attention to patients' specific needs
RES3	Understanding of the specific requirements of patients and patient parties
RES4	Keeping patients informed about when services will be performed
RES5	Promptness of response of employees of the healthcare organisation to any request or complaint
RES6	Capability of response in case of delayed or cancelled services
ASS1	Sincerity and patience in resolving patients' and patients' parties' problems
ASS2	Probability of wrong treatment, death rate

(Table 3.1 continued)

(*Table 3.1 continued*)

ASS3	Safety performance of healthcare organisations
ASS4	Knowledgeable and skilful provision of services
ASS5	Sincere and responsive attitude to patient and patients' party complaints
ASS6	Capacity of staff to instil confidence in patients
ASS7	Capacity of staff to be consistently courteous
ASS8	Presence of knowledgeable employees to answer patients' questions
EMP1	Convenient scheduling for in-patient and out-patient treatment
EMP2	Spontaneous care and concern for patients' needs
EMP3	Frequent service rounds by physicians and staff
EMP4	Possession of a sound loyalty programme to recognise patients as frequent clients
EMP5	Availability of sound treatment packages
EMP6	Availability of other services such as car/ambulance rentals, hiring special attendants/nurses, staying facilities in emergency, 24-hour medical shops, hotels and canteens, washing services on payment, medical insurance, etc.
TEC1	The organisation was successful in curing a patient.
TEC2	Physicians and staff have knowledge and skills.
TEC3	It is a reliable organisation.
IMA1	It is a successful healthcare organisation.
IMA2	It has modern medical equipment and treatment facilities.
IMA3	The organisation has a good reputation.
IMA4	It is sincere with patients.
IMA5	Choose one logo for the organisation which is close to the organisational image.

Source: Parasuraman (1988).

regarding how much improvement is required in service quality in order to achieve patient satisfaction in the future. This research report will guide the government in measuring the level of quality provided by both private and government hospitals and primary healthcare centres.

In future extensions of its scope, this research will utilise multiple data sources, including medical records, patient surveys and administrative data, which may help provide valuable contributions to the growing field of health services.

—

References

AHA (American Hospital Association) Board of Trustees (1992). 'A Patients' Bill of Rights', AHA Management Advisory, Catalog No. 157759, AHA, Chicago.

Babakus, E., and G. W. Boller (1992). 'An Empirical Assessment of the SERVQUAL Scale', *Journal of Business Research*, vol. 24, pp. 253–68.

Brown, S., and T. A. Swartz (1989). 'A Gap Analysis of Professional Service Quality', *Journal of Marketing*, vol. 53, pp. 92–108.

Carman, J. M. (1990). 'Consumer Perceptions of Service Quality: An Assessment of the SERVQUAL Dimensions', *Journal of Retailing*, vol. 66, no. 1, pp. 33–55.

Croze, C. (1994). 'Network Collaboration Can Produce Integrated Care', *Behavioral Health Care Tomorrow*, vol. 3, no. 6, pp. 41, 44–46.

Gronroos, C. (1988). 'Service Quality: The Six Criteria of Good Perceived Service Quality', *Review of Business*, vol. 9, no. 3, pp. 10–13.

Lehtinen, U., and J. R. Lehtinen (1982). 'Service Quality: A Study of Quality Dimensions', unpublished working paper, Service Management Institute, Helsinki.

Oliver, K. A., M. Johnsen and L. Samberg (1999). 'Consumer Satisfaction and Outcomes', Report on Maryland Public Mental Health System, Maryland.

Oliver, R. L., and J. E. Swan (1989). 'Consumer Perceptions of Interpersonal Equity and Satisfaction in Transaction: A Fields Survey Approach', *Journal of Marketing*, vol. 53, pp. 21–35.

Parasuraman, A., V. A. Zeithaml and L. L. Berry (1985). 'A Conceptual Model of Service Quality and Its Implications for Future Research', *Journal of Marketing*, vol. 49, pp. 41–50.

Parasuraman, A., V. A. Zeithaml and L. L. Berry (1988). 'SERVQUAL: A Multiple Item Scale for Measuring Consumer Perception of Service Quality', *Journal of Retailing*, vol. 64, pp. 12–40.

Richard, M. D., and A. W. Allaway (1993). 'Service Quality Attributes and Choice Behavior', *Journal of Service Marketing*, vol. 17, no. 1, pp. 59–68.

Strassar, S., and S. Scheweikhart (1994). *Health Information Management*, Aspen Publishing.

Swartz, T. A., and S. W. Brown (1989). 'Consumer and Provider Expectations and Experiences Evaluating Professional Service Quality', *Journal of the Academy of Marketing Science*, vol. 17, no. 2, pp. 189–95.

4

Challenges to E-Governance Projects in Public Healthcare in India

Aritra Pal, Arunabha Biswas and J. Ajith Kumar

◻

For decades, public health in India has been a significant challenge to its governments. Although the period since 1980 has seen a tremendous improvement in Indian healthcare, several challenges remain. The World Bank Annual Report in 2001 (World Bank 2001) revealed that compared to other developing nations, infant mortality and morbidity in India were significantly greater. Further, a report by the Confederation of Indian Industry and McKinsey (CII and McKinsey & Co. 2002) revealed that only about 15 per cent of the Indian population was covered by some type of insurance. As a result, access to healthcare has remained out of reach for many.

Modern healthcare facilities are prevalent mostly in urban areas, while rural penetration is relatively shallow. A case study performed at the Harvard Business School (Oberholzer-Gee et al. 2007) revealed that the quality of government-provided care in India, while more affordable than private services, was often wanting. The study quotes Dr Atul Gawande, a surgeon at Boston's Brigham and Women's Hospital, who describes a visit to a government-run hospital in India:

> The examining rooms . . . are ovens in the heat of the summer. The paint flakes off the walls in jagged strips. The sinks are stained brown and the faucets don't work. . . . each room has a crowd of four, six, sometimes eight patients jockeying for attention. . . . I asked people everywhere what they did when they had a serious health problem. All of them from villagers to the government doctors themselves told me that, if there was any way they could, they went to a private hospital, though the government does not pay for it . . . even the Prime Minister does not go to his government's hospitals.

These reports not only point to poor levels of public healthcare in India, but also underscore a stark urban–rural divide in the public health scenario in the country. From another perspective, however, the lack of investment in rural areas along with high infrastructural costs has provided opportunities to invoke the use of information and communication technology (ICT) to improve the state of rural Indian healthcare. For example, it is now possible for relevant data and information about a patient to be transferred to a geographically distant doctor who can diagnose the problem and offer a prescription in real time, without ever physically meeting the patient. Encouraged by such possibilities, the central government, as well as various state governments in India, along with assistance from non-governmental organisations (NGOs) and players in the private sector, have taken initiatives to bring doctors and patients closer, reduce the urban–rural healthcare gap, and raise the overall level of healthcare services in the country.

However, these efforts have not been devoid of risks and challenges. This chapter presents an exploratory study that sought to unravel the challenges faced by government-led public e-health projects in India and certain African countries, and, based on the findings, to build a generic framework of potential risks and challenges that any e-health project faces. We felt that such a framework can guide the development of assessment tools for planners and implementers of e-health projects in India and countries with similar contextual settings.

Methodology

The exploration began with a search for pertinent literature (papers in journals, news articles and reports) on e-governance projects in the domain of public health. Among several such projects that find mention in the literature, 15 public health e-governance projects were shortlisted for deeper examination. The shortlisting was guided by: the adequacy of the information available on the project, the mention and/or description of at least one challenge or risk faced by the project, and the geographical context of the project. The final criterion was applied since findings from countries that have similar economic, climatic and socio-economic conditions as India might reveal risks and challenges similar to those found in the Indian subcontinent. As a result, the 15 projects selected were from India, South Africa, Nigeria, Senegal and Ethiopia, with nearly 71 per cent of these originating in India (see Table 4.1). A systematic examination of the shortlisted

Table 4.1 Projects Shortlisted for the Study

S. No.	Project	Country	Mission
1	DRISHTEE	India	Online distance medical diagnosis and consultancy from reputed specialised doctors to rural, poor people to bring effective healthcare to their doorsteps at reduced costs
2	Family Welfare and Health Information Monitoring System (FHIMS)	India(Andhra Pradesh)	To offer a comprehensive software solution for computerising the operations of the Department of Health and Family Welfare
3	Healthcare Information Systems (HIS)	India	Automation of healthcare and dissemination of health-related knowledge to rural people
4	Integrated Disease Surveillance Project (IDSP)	India	To facilitate timely and effective public health actions with respect to communicable and non-communicable diseases, to improve the efficiency of the existing surveillance activities and to facilitate sharing of relevant information
5	India Healthcare (IHC)	India(Rajasthan)	Empowering the village healthcare worker to provide timely care and information
6	Maternity system (CRADLE)	South Africa	Reducing maternal and infant mortality and improving the health of mothers and babies
7	MINPHIS	Nigeria	The reports include patient status, medical history and admissions plus indicators like length of stay per patient, discharge summaries, mortality and morbidity data, and operations

(*Table 4.1 continued*)

(*Table 4.1 continued*)

8	Networking Community Health Centres (CHCs)	South Africa	To integrate the CHCs and network them with other healthcare systems to provide accurate information for health workers
9	Teleclinic	India	Healthcare access to rural masses
10	Telemedicine (north-east [NE])	India	Use of electronic ICTs to provide and support healthcare when distance separates the participants
11	Telemedicine (West Bengal [WB])	India	Use of electronic ICTs to provide and support healthcare when distance separates the participants
12	Telemedicine (Himachal Pradesh [HP])	India	Medical consultation in remote rural areas
13	Teleophthalmology	India	Making eye care services accessible to everyone; eye awareness programmes; training teachers for vision screening programme; comprehensive eye examination in rural areas at patients' doorsteps; and dispensing spectacles at nominal cost
14	WOREDA	Ethiopia	To disseminate healthcare information to all levels of government through internet protocol based services.
15	Yashaswini	India	Free consultations, diagnostics at discounted rates, covering over 1,700 types of operations on the stomach, brain, gall bladder, spine, bones, kidneys and heart

Source: Prepared by the authors.

literature was then done to identify the challenges and risks mentioned, and to understand their impacts on their respective projects. A master list of the challenges was made, followed by a consolidation on the basis of overlaps and similarities between challenges. A total of 23 challenges were finally classified into five categories: technological, socio-economic, human resource, operational and strategic, and are presented in Figure 4.1. Table 4.2 provides a mapping of each specific project to the various challenges faced.

Figure 4.1 Types of Challenges Faced by E-Governance Projects in Public Health

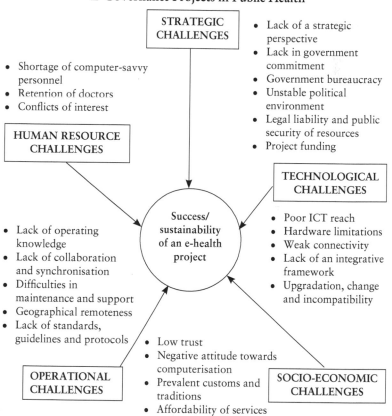

STRATEGIC CHALLENGES
- Lack of a strategic perspective
- Lack in government commitment
- Government bureaucracy
- Unstable political environment
- Legal liability and public security of resources
- Project funding

HUMAN RESOURCE CHALLENGES
- Shortage of computer-savvy personnel
- Retention of doctors
- Conflicts of interest

OPERATIONAL CHALLENGES
- Lack of operating knowledge
- Lack of collaboration and synchronisation
- Difficulties in maintenance and support
- Geographical remoteness
- Lack of standards, guidelines and protocols

TECHNOLOGICAL CHALLENGES
- Poor ICT reach
- Hardware limitations
- Weak connectivity
- Lack of an integrative framework
- Upgradation, change and incompatibility

SOCIO-ECONOMIC CHALLENGES
- Low trust
- Negative attitude towards computerisation
- Prevalent customs and traditions
- Affordability of services

Success/ sustainability of an e-health project

Source: Prepared by the authors.

Table 4.2 Identification of the Types of Challenges Faced by Various Projects

	DRISHTEE	EHIMS	HIS	IDSP	IHC	CRADLE	MINPHIS	Networking CHCs	Teleclinic	Telemedicine (NE)	Telemedicine (WB)	Telemedicine (HP)	Teleophthalmology	WOREDA	Yashaswini
Technological challenges															
Poor ICT reach	✓					✓		✓				✓	✓	✓	
Hardware limitations	✓											✓			
Weak connectivity												✓			
Lack of an integrative framework					✓							✓	✓		
Upgradation, change and incompatibility						✓			✓	✓	✓				
Socio-economic challenges															
Low trust					✓	✓									
Negative attitude towards computerisation		✓										✓			
Prevalent customs and traditions				✓		✓			✓						
Affordability of services															
Human resource challenges															

Shortage of computer-savvy personnel

Retention of doctors

Conflicts of interest

Operational challenges

Lack of operating knowledge

Lack of collaboration and synchronisation

Difficulties in maintenance and support

Geographical remoteness

Lack of standards, guidelines and protocols

Strategic challenges

Lack of a strategic perspective

Lack in government commitment

Government bureaucracy

Unstable political environment

Legal liability and public security of resources

Project funding

Source: Prepared by the authors.

The Challenges

While different challenges manifested themselves differently across the projects, the frequency of occurrence, as well as the influence, of each challenge too varied across projects. Some challenges occurred more frequently than others, while some had relatively more influence on the projects than others. To gain more insight, an assessment was made using a 5-point Likert scale of the impacts of the challenges on the projects, based entirely on the information found, and is presented in Table 4.3. A rating of '5' indicates that the challenge posed a major hurdle to the project, while '1' denotes that either this challenge was hardly felt in the project or was not mentioned at all in the literature found. An overall score was computed for each challenge by adding up the ratings obtained by that challenge across projects, to discern the relative impacts of the respective challenges.[1] It was found that operational, strategic and technological challenges were the most, while socio-economic and human resources challenges were the least, influential. In the next section, the different challenges and their driving factors are explored in more detail.

Table 4.3 Project-wise Assessment of the Challenges

Project	Technological	Socio-economic	Operational	Human Resource	Strategic
DRISHTEE	4	3	4	1	4
FHIMS	4	4	4	1	5
HIS	1	1	4	4	3
IDSP	2	5	2	1	1
IHC	2	4	5	2	1
CRADLE	2	5	2	1	1
MINPHIS	1	1	1	5	4
Networking CHCs	4	2	3	3	3
Teleclinic	3	1	4	1	5
Telemedicine (NE)	4	1	3	4	4
Telemedicine (WB)	4	1	4	5	3
Telemedicine (HP)	5	1	4	3	3
Teleophthalmology	5	3	2	2	2
WOREDA	4	2	3	4	4
Yashaswini	1	1	3	1	4
Overall score	46	35	48	38	47

Technological Challenges

As e-governance health projects are heavily dependent on the use of ICT for carrying out their operations, it is not surprising that technological challenges played a significant role in the success and sustainability of these projects. Nearly 72 per cent of the projects studied faced technological challenges in some form or the other. In the healthcare context, technology gains paramount importance particularly when information processing and transfer has to be achieved in real time with minimal delay. In some cases, delays can lead to loss of life or permanent impairment. Technological challenges can arise in the following ways.

Poor ICT Reach

The telemedicine project in West Bengal was challenged right at the outset by the poor reach of ICT in the targeted areas as reported on the Department of Administrative Reforms and Public Grievances (DARPG) website (see Shukla and Maity 2006). Developing countries in general are handicapped by a low internet penetration, particularly in rural areas. As per the statistics available on the Internet World Stats website, the current internet penetration in India is about 15.8 per cent;[2] this figure is much lower in rural areas. When compared with penetration rates of greater than 50 per cent in developed nations as given on the same website, it is easy to see why e-healthcare in India would be significantly up against this challenge. The costs of basic elements such as personal computers, printers, modems, power stabilisers and licensed software can make it difficult to justify their use only for offering government-related information. From the perspective of kiosk operators, through whom e-health projects are often rolled out in rural areas, the return on such investments can be too low, and, to be profitable, alternative revenue-generating streams may be necessary.

Hardware Limitations

The telemedicine projects, specifically those implemented in the north-eastern states of India and in West Bengal, faced problems due to capacity constraints (Sood and Bhatia 2005). The demand for services increased almost exponentially once projects found acceptability among the masses, but capacity was a limitation. Hardware capacity, e.g., data storage and network bandwidth capacity, should be chosen such that the system remains scalable in the face of high demand in the future. Hence, it may be necessary to have the correct demand estimation in place during the implementation stage. Otherwise, data crashes, network failures and ultimately systemic breakdowns can result, entailing loss of confidence among the masses.

Weak Connectivity

Healthcare projects, particularly those that involve life-critical activities and can be of high priority, require trouble-free and smooth connectivity through dedicated channels. The telemedicine projects in India (Sood and Bhatia 2005) and the CRADLE project in South Africa (Mars and Seebregts 2008), suffered frequent data losses and even data crashes at peak times due to intermittent connectivity. In rural India, achieving continuous connectivity, due to the poor infrastructure, is one of the most common problems faced. Low bandwidth can make the system incapable of handling the extra load in times of peak demand, which can eventually lead to network crashes and the entire system going defunct.

Lack of an Integrative Framework

Normally, when two systems are connected, a little functionality is lost from each, according to Lau (2003). The degree of functionality lost is directly proportional to the number of systems connected. The high diversity of healthcare organisations, coupled with the heterogeneity of information systems, has meant that integration has and may continue to be a problem area in the future unless due care is taken. The HIS project faced this problem. Since the project involved many different agencies and the healthcare departments of the various states across India, integration of these independent entities was complex and caused unnecessary delays in the implementation of the project. In reality, true integration is still a rare occurrence. To alleviate this problem, a technological framework and establishment of common rules and standards to connect various systems may be required. Handling a diversity of information and communication systems thus introduces other costs to the project.

Upgradation, Change and Incompatibility

Compatibility can play a significant role in the acceptability of healthcare projects. Consider the example of the WOREDA health-care project in Ethiopia (see UN 2011). Although the government introduced electronic healthcare cards for the citizens, the project's popularity was quite low due to the lack of private clinics and facilities that actually accepted the card for transactions with consumers. Thus, the card (and eventually, the project) was perceived as being of low value.

The rapid appearance of new versions of software and hardware in the market rapidly leads to a multiplicity in the types of technology and software systems used for front-end as well as back-end operations. This multiplicity may give rise to various incompatibilities, which, if neglected, can lead to the creation of watertight systems that cannot communicate with each other. Acceptability problems may also arise when trying to decide upon a new standard that is yet to be accepted by the market. Hence, there is a need for unification and standardisation of hardware, software and applications for the various systems, and it is preferable to use standard instead of custom-made software for greater acceptability. Technology upgradation and change also necessitates doctors and staff to adjust to these changes, but work pressures, time constraints and inherent aversion to the digitisation can deter change.

Socio-economic Challenges

The findings revealed that e-health services can be challenged by prevailing socio-economic conditions. Sometimes, even after service facilities are set up and doctors are available, people in remote locations may not be willing to accept their services. In some cases, on-field staff in remote locations reported unacceptability as a major challenge to their work. One of the projects faced instances of hindrance and disturbance from the locals. Of the 15 projects studied, 6 projects (40 per cent) faced some degree of this challenge, which can arise in different ways.

Low Trust

In some projects, local people did not treat the health workers well. When the root cause for this was analysed, it was found that health workers preached against the locals' beliefs. For example, while locals believed that having more children was good, health workers preached just the opposite. This caused conflict, and subsequently health workers faced difficulties in mingling with the locals. The lack of education among the rural population in India can be seen as playing truant here. Both the teleophthalmology as well as the IHC projects (Graves and Reddy 2000) faced this problem. The Indianchild.com website notes:

> The integration of health services with family planning programmes often causes the local population to perceive the primary health centers as hostile to their traditional preference for large families. Therefore, primary health centers often play an adversarial role in local efforts to implement national health policies.[3]

Often, the lack of infrastructural frameworks, including education, is one of the major reasons why projects face problems at the grassroots. This is also one of the reasons that there is a health awareness divide.

Negative Attitude towards Computerisation

One of the challenges evident from the FHIMS project was that parallel manual systems continued, as all the reports required could not be generated with FHIMS itself.[4] The usage of the system has been well below its expected levels, and owing to psychological discomfort with technology, people have displayed low motivation to use the system. It has been found that in some cases, the doctors and staff were reluctant to work with the latest information technology (IT) gadgets. Often, the doctors themselves were not very aware of e-healthcare. Sometimes, doctors viewed telemedicine as an additional burden, an extra workload. Due to a 'technology-averse' mindset, doctors often wanted the technical staff to operate the instruments, instead of doing it themselves.

Prevalent Customs and Traditions

The Integrated Disease Surveillance Project faced challenges of a different type — prevalent customs, traditions, norms and superstitions.[5]

In many parts of India, particularly rural India, the joint family system exists even today. In such families, most major decisions are made by the head of the family, and followed by the others with almost no questioning. Thus, traditional means of treatment such as homemade remedies often take precedence over modern medicine. Gender bias is also prevalent. While treatment for men is sought very promptly when they fall sick, women are not given the same importance. In fact, such delays often lead to the deterioration of the health conditions of women. Interestingly, the IDSP describes some instances where the tribal population treats men and women as equal, and decisions are made jointly; however, these cases are few and far between.

It was also found that in some places, tribals and villagers did not consider sickness as a medical problem. Having deep faith in old wisdom and beliefs, some perceived disease as a curse from God, and believed that making offerings and sacrifices at the local temple was the remedy. Such offerings ranged from fruits and flowers to even liquor, chicken and goat. In other places, tribals sought homemade remedies as the first resort. If the symptoms didn't subside, they sought the help of traditional healers (or quacks), rather than modern doctors. This was also because the tribal population did not entirely trust the credibility of the health system. They perceived that the public healthcare system was not sufficiently concerned about economically backward people, and did not provide adequate treatment.

Affordability of Services

An important question that needs to be asked before an e-healthcare project is launched is: can the target population afford the services we intend to provide, at the rate at which we can price it? If the services are not affordable by a large section of the people they are intended for, the investments and effort may be wasted. Antony and Laxmaiah (2008) note that post-independence, poverty reduction has been a primary focus in India. Despite significant progress, 260 million are still below the poverty line, and this population contributes one-fourth of the world's poor.

In the case of the teleclinic project that was carried out in the Bundelkhand region of Madhya Pradesh in India, the masses (for whom the project was developed) had difficulties in affording the services, leading to a mismatch between the intention and the actual implementation. Consequently, the sustainability of the project was at stake. At the core of the problem was a weak and unsustainable revenue model, which had not clearly accounted for how telemedicine consultants would be paid; indeed such problems were also faced by the teleophthalmology project (Vision 2020 2006). To overcome such problems, the Nkoranza Community Health Financing Scheme has been developed in Ghana to finance the entire e-health scheme via membership.

Human Resource Challenges

As with any management initiative, providing appropriate manpower is a primary concern in the success of e-healthcare projects, for it is the people who ultimately make things happen. For a project to be successful, it needs trained doctors, dedicated support staff, their willingness and enthusiasm, their ability to take on the excess load when needed, and their eagerness to serve the masses. Inadequate manpower can lead the project to jeopardy. Lack of ownership, lack of direction, misalignment of individual objectives with the overall goals and the lack of technical skills were among the major findings that came out in the study. The conflicting priorities of various stakeholders and their individual aims and aspirations made some projects resemble a ship being propelled simultaneously in different directions. Eight of the 15 projects that were studied (53 per cent) experienced challenges related to manpower.

Shortage of Computer-Savvy Personnel

In the CRADLE project of South Africa ((Mars and Seebregts 2008), the computer literacy rate and the absence of computer terminologies in various languages was a major cause of concern. This often led to the inability to comprehend computer language, despite being considered literate, resulting in problems with the usability of the system. Low levels of computer literacy caused a dearth of available manpower during the selection of on-field operators, while existing staff members had little exposure to computers during their basic training and school education. This was also partly due to the differences between the education systems in urban and rural areas. Among doctors too, there was a digital bar. Some doctors did well, but others were averse to the use of computers. Their curriculum did not have any computer literacy course. As a result, the nodal centres needed to have a helper (technician) to help the doctor out. Although attempts were made to train the support staff gradually, the responses from the support staff were not very encouraging, and a sense of negativism regarding computerisation prevailed among public health officials.

Retention of Doctors

In the telemedicine project (Bhatia n.d.), retention of doctors was a significant challenge, revealing how difficult it was to retain doctors in rural areas. From the perspective of doctors, there was a risk of becoming professionally isolated and even obsolete. Monetary incentives offered to doctors were not sufficient to motivate them to work in rural areas, as the socio-economic conditions and the existing infrastructure proved to be major obstacles. According to Mishra et al. (2007), 75 per cent of qualified consulting doctors practise in urban centres and 23 per cent in semi-urban areas, and only 2 per cent in rural areas. On the other hand, a majority of the patients come from rural areas. Of late, the Government of India has been trying to send interns to the village masses by making internship in rural areas mandatory, giving suitable incentives to the interns, but these efforts are yet to bear fruit.

Conflict of Interests

Sometimes, different stakeholders in a project may view the project differently. This was observed in the MINPHIS project (Afolabi 2004). While some viewed the project as a research activity, others saw it as a cash cow, and yet others saw it as a stepping stone to creating regional centres of excellence and training. These differences led to conflicts of interest and, being pulled in different directions, the aim of the project was diluted.

Operational Challenges

Operational challenges arise for various reasons, one of them being a faulty approach taken to implementing and running the project. The major source of such problems is the lack of detailed planning in the pre-implementation phase, when these problems are invisible, but which manifest themselves during the implementation and post-implementation phases. Of the different projects studied, almost 57 per cent faced operational challenges in one form or the other. The involvement of several actors in healthcare projects, like doctors, midwife nurses, government agencies and private players, made operational challenges quite frequent in such projects. Operational challenges are of higher complexity than technological and financial challenges. Five ways in which operational challenges arise were identified.

Lack of Operating Knowledge

This is a major issue for various organisations that are involved in the implementation and post-implementation phases of a project. As most of the healthcare projects are implemented in the interior rural regions, the working teams belonging to the various consultancy and technological firms may not be well oriented to working in such environments. Problems such as non-communicability due to language differences tend to inhibit the full understanding of the processes behind the work being performed in those regions. Limited global experience in handling such projects can also add to the misery. For example, according to Graves and Reddy (2000), the India Healthcare pilot project's failures in Rajasthan could be attributed to the limited experience of the engineering teams from Apple Inc. and CMC Ltd in healthcare projects, and their almost complete lack of experience in comprehending the way healthcare supervision is carried out by auxiliary midwives in rural Rajasthan. Organisations with proper experience in handling such projects and a thorough operational knowledge of the project along with information about the rural area and its populace are imperatives for the success of such projects.

Lack of Collaboration and Synchronisation

Since e-governance projects are generally huge in terms of both scale and scope, they entail the involvement of multiple organisations and stakeholders, both public and private, before and after their implementation. There is bound to be a need for intelligent collaboration among these stakeholders. Further, synchronisation of communication can become critical to the success of the project. However, high levels of complexity can make this very difficult. Collaboration and synchronisation difficulties also arise due to reasons such as time differences, differing communicational styles, organisation-specific infrastructure differences, different degrees of participation in the projects, privacy and security concerns restricting the sharing of data between different government departments, and differences in interests, expectations and responsibilities. For example, the tele-medicine project in West Bengal, as cited on the DARPG website, struggled due to a lack of coordination with referral centres to fix a mutually convenient tele-consultation. In another case, Apple and CMC, partners in the IHC project in Rajasthan, differed starkly from each other in size, working culture, management styles and the types of projects handled, and this led to several problems as discussed by Graves and Reddy (2000). The end result — failure of the entire project.

Difficulty in Maintenance and Support

Occurring in the post-implementation phase, these challenges can deter the normal working of the system. Small problems such as bugs, unaddressed system errors, intermittent power supply and low maintainability can bring the entire system to a halt. This can be a serious concern in the health domain, where continuous connectivity and real-time processing of data are necessary. For example, in the IHC project in Rajasthan, which involved carrying portable digital diaries to interior rural areas for the collection and transmission of information, the battery life was not sufficient for the device as noted by Graves and Reddy (2000). The batteries were also expensive as well as cumbersome to carry and change. Solar panels, a solution to this problem, required a huge budget and time, hence the entire project was eventually declared infeasible and shelved.

Geographical Remoteness

Geographical remoteness can induce risks and costs into a project, particularly in the context of rural healthcare. All the 15 health projects studied were rural projects. Most future projects in India will also be in rural regions as governments seek to remove the digital divide and aim for inclusive growth. Generally, geographical remoteness spawns challenges of accessibility, transportation and extreme weather conditions in the interior parts of the country. In the IHC project studied, extreme weather conditions due to sand and heat in the desert affected the message pad's serial port and screen, and the entire structure of the electronic device had to be changed, according to Graves and Reddy (2000).

Lack of Standards, Guidelines and Protocols

The incorporation of multipurpose telemedicine standards to meet the needs of the diverse user groups at different levels of the hierarchy acts as a barrier to the effective functioning of the projects. Both the pan-India and the West Bengal–specific telemedicine projects, as mentioned by Bedi (2003) and by Sood and Bhatia (2005), were plagued by this problem. The inability of the various departments to communicate with each other obstructs the seamless delivery of services. Frameworks and common standards can increase collaboration and help in keeping the e-government activity aligned on the agendas of public administration.

The lack of guidelines and protocols can also pose a threat to the privacy and security of citizens' data and transactions with the government. In turn, this can create citizens' lack of confidence in the government and result in the dumping of the services by the citizens. Having common guidelines and protocols in place is a necessary, but not sufficient, condition for achieving collaboration. The teleophthalmology project in Senegal, aimed at making specialised eye health available in rural zones, faced this problem (Colomé et al. 2009).

Strategic Challenges

E-governance, as the name suggests, involves the government as the primary stakeholder, and the locus of control for implementing the projects lies with it. In certain cases, there is a lack of flexibility in the government framework which deters the smooth implementation and operation of the e-governance projects and gives rise to external barriers. Almost 29 per cent of the healthcare projects studied faced this type of a barrier. These challenges can arise in six different forms.

Lack of a Strategic Perspective

A strategic perspective on a project must consider all its dimensions instead of just some. Sometimes, however, this perspective may be lacking. For example, in the CHC project in South Africa, as described by Lemon et al. (2006), and in healthcare projects in Nigeria (Afolabi 2004), the primary focus was on ICT aspects, and these projects were considered mainly to be merely shifts from manual ways of working to automated versions. Little attention was paid to end-customer requirements and the corresponding process improvements that were needed. The fact that rural people are hard pressed to articulate their expectations of services from the government complicates this further. A clear understanding of the overall mission of the project and its relevance to all the stakeholders is required during the planning phase itself. Subordinating the strategic perspective to a narrower one is a major cause of failure of projects after they have been implemented, thus draining money and effort.

Lack in Government Commitment

The government is expected to be a major promoter of public health projects, particularly in developing countries such as India; hence the lack of government commitment can be a major barrier for project success. Sometimes, indifference on the part of government agencies to actively participate in running the project can stall or defuse a project. For example, in the WOREDA project in Ethiopia, which involved disseminating healthcare information to all levels of the government, it was observed that there was a significant delay in getting permission from various government departments (UN 2011). Often, before launching a major e-governance project, small pilot projects are run for feasibility studies, and sometimes the government agencies, considering such pilot projects to be mere research exercises, do not take them seriously. This greatly undermines the future chances of the main project being implemented. Lau (2003) states that in the current public governance framework, government agencies work in silos, thus inhibiting collaboration and information sharing among others. This translates into agencies not being able to determine properly what is required of them, resulting in a lower level of commitment and willingness to invest in such projects.

Government Bureaucracy

In some cases, government high-handedness and adherence to a top–down approach has led to projects being abandoned by workers situated at lower rungs in the hierarchy. Even after successful planning and implementation, projects sometimes failed to achieve active participation and involvement at the operational level due to a lackadaisical attitude by the staff. According to Bedi (2003), in the pan-India telemedicine project, for example, it was noted that parallel manual systems coexisted with the automated systems. At the end of the day, it is the staff and the people in the lower rungs of management who look after daily operations, and in this sense, the ultimate power rests with them.

Unstable Political Environment

This continues to be a challenge for e-governance projects in developing and underdeveloped nations. Generally, e-governance projects, being government projects, are initiated by a particular political party forming the government. Owing to frequent changes of ruling parties in unstable political situations, projects tend to suffer by losing the attention and funds they received earlier from the party that promoted them. An example of this is Senegal's teleophthalmology project, as described by Colomé et al. (2009), which almost went to the verge of being called off by the new government. Such situations can sometimes lead to the shelving of some projects, with initial costs going down as sunk costs.

Legal Liabilities and Public Security of Resources

Generally, IT-related laws are enforced for security and confidentiality reasons, but the complexity of such laws can impede the sharing of data across different agencies. Moreover, regulatory guidance also poses challenges to e-governance coordinators; e.g., accountability rules, which are framed to ensure responsible use of public resources by making people more accountable, can inhibit collaboration in the case of shared projects. According to Lau (2003), removing the legal and technological barriers can help in achieving economies of scale by adopting a whole-of-government approach and reducing disparate legacy systems.

Project Funding

Three financing models were prevalent in the projects studied. While some projects were fully government-funded, others were fully sponsored by private parties and NGOs. A hybrid model was followed by other projects, wherein the government and private parties came together under public–private partnerships. Timely availability of funds was a hurdle faced by some of the e-health projects, and the lack of funds also led to questioning the sustainability of some of the projects. For example, the MINPHIS project in Nigeria (Afolabi 2004) was up against a shortage of funds: the more time this project took, the more its costs increased. However, it is not uncommon for public health e-governance projects to attract external funding, though funding was not a major problem in many projects.

Thus, this section has presented a classification of the various challenges and the factors that underlie them, based on the information found during the study.

Conclusion

This chapter presents findings from an exploratory study based on publicly available information, to provide a glimpse into the variety of potential challenges that a typical e-governance project in public healthcare can face. Twenty-three different challenges were categorised into five types — technological, socio-economic, human resource, operational and strategic. Although the study is based on secondary information, it nevertheless affirms that a multidimensional perspective needs to be adopted in tackling the problem of setting up and running e-health systems in the country. As Table 4.3 reveals, no project faces just one type of challenge, and no challenge manifests in only one project.

It is also felt that the interactions between the challenges play an important role in determining the success of a project and its sustainability. While a low score on all challenging factors may seem to indicate higher chances of success for a project, the interactions between factors must not be ignored. It is felt that the framework of challenges proposed in this chapter, along with the various factors causing them, can be developed into a useful tool for assessing the risks involved in a project during the conceptualisation, strategising and planning stages. Based on the levels of challenges facing a particular project, appropriate strategies can be pursued. Frameworks such as the one presented in this study can be useful in helping further the initiatives of India's governments in moving towards equitable healthcare in the country.

Care was taken to ensure that only information from reliable sources was used for the analyses done in this study. Yet, in some cases, it is observed that richer and more detailed sources of information could have aided the cause of more rigorous assessment. The data (or information) used in this chapter were taken only from secondary sources. It is felt that a more detailed study based on primary data can provide more insight into the nature of the challenges faced and risks present in public e-health projects in the country.

—

Notes

1. Since a 1–5 rating scale was used and summing was done across 15 projects, the overall score can range between 15 and 75.
2. Internet World Stats, http://www.internetworldstats.com/asia.htm (accessed on 15 February 2015).
3. 'Health Care in India', http://www.indianchild.com/health_care_in_india. htm (accessed on 28 February 2010).
4. 'Documentation on Methodology Used for Providing Support in Implementation of FHIMS Both at the PHC and District (DM&HOs) Levels', http://www.uio.no/studier/emner/matnat/ifi/INF5730/h04/under-visningsmateriale/inf5730-method.pdf (accessed on 28 February 2010).
5. Integrated Disease Surveillance Project, http://idsp.nic.in/ (accessed on 28 February 2010).

References

Afolabi, Adekunle Oluseyi (2004). 'MINPHIS: Improving Patient Data in a Nigerian Hospital', eGovernment for Development, eHealth Case Study No. 3, http://www.egov4dev.org/health/case/minphis.shtml (accessed on 15 February 2015).

Antony, G. M., and A. Laxmaiah (2008). 'Human Development, Poverty, Health and Nutrition Situation in India', *Indian Journal of Medical Research*, vol. 128, pp. 198–205.

Bedi, B. S. (2003). 'Telemedicine in India: Initiatives and Perspective', eHealth 2003: Addressing the Digital Divide, http://www.oldagesolutions.org/publications/bedi_telemedicine_india.pdf (accessed on 11 January 2015).

Bhatia, B. S. (n.d.). 'Telemedicine Network Implementation: Challenges and Issues', http://laico.org/v2020resource/files/telemedicine_challenges.pdf (accessed on 28 February 2010).

CII (Confederation of Indian Industry) and McKinsey & Co. (2002). *Healthcare in India: The Road Ahead*, New Delhi: CII.

Colomé, Josep, Jaume Benseny, Albert Domingo, Sergi Marí, Xavier Caufapé and Rafael Ferreruela (2009). 'Tele-Ophthalmology Eye Health System Deployment in Kolda, Senegal', http://wwwold.i2cat.net/files/Tele-Ophthalmology%20Eye-Health%20 system%20deployment%20in%20Kolda.pdf (accessed on 11 January 2015).

Graves, M., and N. K. Reddy (2000). 'Electronic Support for Rural Healthcare Workers', in *Information and Communication Technology in Development: Cases from India*, edited by S. Bhatnagar and R. Schware, New Delhi, Sage Publications, pp. 35–49.

Lau, E. (2003). 'Challenges for E-Government Development', 5th Global Forum of Reinventing Government, Mexico City, 5 November, http://unpan1.un.org/intradoc/groups/public/documents/un/unpan 012241.pdf (accessed on 12 January 2015).

Lemon, Stephenie C., Jane G. Zapka, Barbara Estabrook and Evan Benjamin (2006). 'Challenges to Research in Urban Community Health Centers', *American Journal of Public Health*, vol. 96, no. 4, pp. 626–28, http:// www.ncbi.nlm.nih.gov/pmc/articles/PMC1470532/ (accessed on 12 January 2015).

Mars, Maurice, and Chris Seebregts (2008). 'Country Case Study for e-Health South Africa', http://ehealth-connection.org/files/resources/ County%20Case%20Study%20for%20eHealth%20South%20Africa. pdf (accessed on 12 January 2015).

Mishra, S. K., D. Gupta and J. Kaur, J. (2007). 'Telemedicine in India: Initiatives and Vision', Paper presented at the 9th International Conference on e-Health Networking, Application & Services, Taipei, Taiwan, 19–22 June, http://www.stbmi.ac.in/matter/international%20 pub/34_Telemedicine%20in%20India%20%20Initiatives%20and%20 vision.pdf (accessed on 15 February 2015).

Oberholzer-Gee, F., T. Khanna and C. Knoop (2007). 'Apollo Hospitals — First-World Healthcare at Emerging-Market Prices', Harvard Business School Case 9-706-440, October.

Shukla, Rajendra S., and J. N. Maity (2006). 'Telemedicine Projects in West Bengal', darpg.nic.in/darpgwebsite_cms/Document/file/telemedicine.ppt (accessed on 12 January 2015).

Sood, S. P., and J. S. Bhatia (2005). 'Development of Telemedicine Technology in India: "Sanjeevani" — An Integrated Telemedicine Application', *Journal of Postgraduate Medicine*, vol. 51, no. 4, pp. 308–11, http://www.ncbi.nlm.nih.gov/pubmed/16388174 (accessed on 15 February 2015).

UN (United Nations) (2011). 'United Nations Report: Ten-Year Appraisal and Review of the Implementation of the Brussels Programme of Action for the Least Developed Countries for the Decade 2001–2010', Paper presented at the Fourth United Nations Conference on the Least Developed Countries, Geneva, 4–29 July, http://unohrlls.org/UserFiles/File/LDC%20Documents/Reports/A-66-66.pdf (accessed 15 February 2015).

Vision 2020 (2006). Tele-ophthalmology, *Sitenews* vol. 3, no. 9, September, http://www.v2020eresource.org/newsitenews.aspx?tpath=news92006 (accessed 15 February 2015).

World Bank (2001). *Year in Review*. Washington, D.C.: World Bank, http://documents.worldbank.org/curated/en/2001/01/2089130/world-bank-annual-report-2001-year-review (accessed on 15 February 2015).

5

The Role of NGOs in Creating Participatory Dialogic Praxis for Community-Based Mental Healthcare

Reflections from Field Experiences at NAMI India

Maheswar Satpathy

◼

The issues of mental health and related care have been ignored in a rapidly developing country like India.[1] Lack of adequate profession-ally trained specialists and almost non-existent institutionalised forms of care have created an anomalous situation. Non-governmental organisations (NGOs) have been engaged in the development of India for years, but only recently has mental health been added to their agenda. This chapter discusses the role of emerging NGOs in a radical participatory dialogic praxis with communities through various communicative new media technologies like information and communication technology (ICT) innovations. The veracity of the assumption regarding the efficacy of these organisations is substanti-ated through experiential insights gained from the Nodal Association on Mental Illness (NAMI) India, a partner of the National Alliance on Mental Illness, USA.

Mental illness — the very phrase conjures up images of forlorn loved ones or frenzied, unkempt people lurking on sidewalks and in dark alleys, talking to themselves, lost in a world of their own. Myths about mental illness abound, and the statistics of its incidence and impact on our common humanity are astounding. Scientific break-throughs hold the promise of recovery, but are unknown and hardly accessible to a largely illiterate and developing society full of preju-dices towards people with mental illnesses. Ironically, in spite of large claims about discoveries in the field of mental healthcare, stigma entraps people with mental illness and endangers their lives. Several issues which have been perennially associated with the concept of mental illness have not changed despite years of struggle and activism. Questions have been raised that mental healthcare in India is in a dilapidated condition, and it is often lamented that the available services seem punitive rather than palliative or curative. The issue is that after years of emergence and initiation of mental healthcare in India, it has not made any significant progress.

In most countries, particularly low- and middle-income countries, mental health services are severely short of resources — both human and financial. Of the healthcare resources available, most are currently spent on the specialised treatment and care of the mentally ill, and to a lesser extent on an integrated mental health system. Instead of providing care in large psychiatric hospitals, countries should integrate mental health into primary healthcare, provide mental healthcare in general hospitals, and develop community-based mental health services. Therefore, mental health promotion necessitates multi-sectorial action, involving a number of government sectors and non-governmental or community-based organisations (CBOs). The focus should be on promoting mental health throughout life, to ensure a healthy start in life for children, and to prevent mental disorders in adults, especially older people.

Why NGOs, and What Can They Do for Community Mental Healthcare?

Over the years, NGOs have been instrumental in spearheading the community-based healthcare movement in India, and this might be one of the reasons behind the meteoric increase in awareness about mental health in the country. Non-governmental organisations have been successful in generating a new momentum in healthcare by creating an urge among common people, as well as specialists, to revamp the healthcare system. The increasing demands for reforms in healthcare and for new forms of healthcare practices, and innovations in services with the assistance of advanced technologies, are an achievement of NGO innovations in both developing as well as developed nations. The merit of these organisations lies in their efficacy in involving the community with the process of planning and execution of healthcare activities by actively working with the community. The focus is always on an integrated project approach rather than a specific need-driven one. They are able to achieve their goals of community involvement by obtaining people's faith and community acceptance for their projects. Today's organisations encourage a high degree of innovation in practices of healthcare and are willing to invest in newer technologies. They believe in practices which reflect a high degree of transparency, accountability and ethical governance. Need-based planning is always strengthened by a preference for team work. As NGOs believe in learning from doing rather than preaching, practices are always orientated towards enabling and facilitation.

Non-governmental organisations adopt several useful and successful practices in order to involve the community and to create a paradigm of participatory engagement to address the larger concerns of society. Some of these are: the practice of result-based management; participatory learning and action; involvement of the community; reaching the unreached and inaccessible areas; human resource development with bottom–up planning, and formation and capacity building of community groups like self-help groups and CBOs. With the help of differential strategic movements, NGOs are able to create appropriate opportunities for the engagement of members of different communities for several causes and concerns.

A few areas where NGOs can work wonders are in the identification and mapping of vulnerable slums, improving access to sanitation and other basic services, enhancing demand for and utilisation of services, building capacities and effective partnerships and convergence. The World Health Organization (WHO) (1991) study group on Community Involvement in Health (CIH) suggested two broad ways of promoting CIH: (a) through awareness and understanding of health and health problems; and (b) through access to information and knowledge about health service programmes and projects. In India, we have emerging organisations which are working on the issue of rehabilitation, prevention and intervention with persons having mental illness. Some of the notable ones are the Schizophrenia Research Foundation India, Ashagram, Samadhan, Paripurnata, and many others which have been noted in a recent book by Patel and Thara (2003). Though success rates vary, they have been instrumental in creating sensitivity towards the issues ailing the system of healthcare in India. Chatterjee et al. (2003) lament the systemic entropy and lack of participation from community members, labelling it as 'patchy', and they ascribe this state of affairs to the non-recognition of communities as stakeholders in systems of care. Hence, they suggest that locally relevant needs can be met only through greater, broad-based mobilisation of communities in order to produce sustainable outcomes in healthcare. Further, emphasis on community involvement is important to achieve broader acceptance of interventions; for this, physical and attitudinal changes have to be brought about through a process of dialogue with local communities (ibid.). This is also supported by the fact that the acceptability of a particular intervention, and its relative effectiveness, depends on the community's participation as integral stakeholders in systems of care.

Why Not Consumers?

The predominant support for the participatory movement or 'learning by doing' of NGOs has caused the traditional expert view, and its imposing stand, to be abandoned. In an interview, when Akila Maheswari, founder president of NAMI India, asked Gayathri Ramaprasad[2] what her suggestions to Indian mental health consumers might be, Ramaprasad expressed deep feelings of dislike for the word 'consumer' itself. She explains, 'I find it inherently discriminatory. I fail to understand why we would want to differentiate people with mental illness from people with all other illnesses. While we refer to them as "patients", we continue to refer to ourselves as "consumers".' She expresses her alternative preference for referring to people with mental illness as 'beautiful minds'!

Participatory Dialogic Praxis and the Role of NGOs

Praxis refers to a process of critical intellectualising and internalising of cultural attributes while allowing for sufficient reflexivity. Dialogue leads to critical reflection, the first step of praxis (Freire 1970), instrumental in developing a cultural and situational consciousness (Dorsey 2010). Through critical reflection and reflexivity, we can decide on and conduct ourselves through appropriate action, which is mostly moderated through a cultural consciousness for determining the appropriateness of the response. Hence, culture and society play an instrumental role in our introspective abilities and the degree of empathy and self-reflexivity we exercise. On a cultural plane, participatory action and exercises in dialogue are expected to develop increased self-reflection and consequently enhanced action. For a 'progressive impact', a move towards radical praxis (Freire 1972a, 1972b; Lather 1986) is suggested in which theory, action and research are intertwined and inseparable, and immersed in the lives of people who are disenfranchised, possibly via more efficacious routes of participation on a community level.

Participatory praxis is committed to mainstreaming the voices of the poor and marginalised sections of society in the process of development. This approach stems from the belief that, for development to be sustainable, the process must be truly participative. With the help of participatory dialogic praxis, NGOs devise practices to enhance the participation of the community in all their endeavours, while at the same time acknowledging that 'participation' is not a technical or a mechanical process that can be realised through the application of a set of static and universal tools and techniques. Rather, it is a political process that requires challenging the existing power structure. Thus, in this approach, the community is not seen as an object but rather as an agent of change. In an attempt to highlight the importance of dialogic partnership between the voluntary organisations and the beneficiaries of care, several researchers (Kagan and Burton 2001) suggest a movement towards a radical praxis, which they prefer to call 'prefigurative praxis':

> [Prefigurative praxis] emphasises the relationship between action research [and practice] and the creation of alternatives to the existing social order. This combined process of social reform and [reflection] enables learning about both the freedom of movement to create progressive social forms and about the constraints the present order imposes. It also creates disseminated 'images of possibility' for a different way of ordering social life (*ibid.*).

Kagan et al. (2000) propose that action, research and theory are inseparably intertwined in complex ways, and deeply immersed in the lives of people who are marginalised, oppressed and dispossessed. There is a need to emphasise a reflexive and historical practice that learns from its past, and challenges the social status quo as well as the status quo within psychology.

Seidman (1986) suggests that a dialectical relationship between people and systems offers a basis for greater dialogue, enabling the true concerns of community members to be voiced. Seidman emphasises that reciprocity and interdependency between individuals and social systems represent a synthesis of community and psychology. Thus, community psychological praxis may provide opportunities for enhancing the creative, determining potential of people (Bhaskar 1989). This type of relationship explores mass consciousness and perceptions towards mental illness, health and well-being, and strives to foster a multi-stakeholder-based participatory action, where no hierarchy or feeling of superiority is allowed to reign in the interactional patterns. This kind of relationship emphasises a true realisation of the needs, concerns, challenges, strengths and opportunities present in a particular community, and takes these as an indicator for designing programmes in consultation with community, which will prove to be optimally beneficial in the long run for collective well-being and act as a catalytic agent for development.

For the optimal realisation of such changes with the active participation of the community, development agencies, whether government, NGOs, CBOs or other civil society organisations, have to define or redefine their roles as facilitators of such participatory processes of development. The process of change reflected in empowering the poor is a political process, which essentially means mainstreaming the marginalised. It challenges the hegemonic power structure and enables people to check, cross-check, analyse and intervene in policies and programmes for development. It may create new institutions; it may break existing ones. Engagement with development agencies and organisations is a critical component of participatory development advocacy. It is a perennial process which adds to our wisdom and learning. Decentralisation of power and local self-governance are the important cornerstones of a truly participatory democracy.

On issues pertaining to how to bring about increased levels of community participation, Bhuyan (2004) suggests a potential tool, i.e., a personally held self-care manual and health record, which he proposes should be designed jointly by the community and professionals. Its first part might contain basic self-care information, and the second part could contain outlines of different personally held health records to be used to record the important health- and disease-related events of an individual. Periodic monitoring and evaluation of the programme may be undertaken by both parties together. The onus of capacity building, institutional strengthening and sustainability lies with NGOs, who can serve as trainers on a variety of topics, e.g., urban vulnerability, behaviour change communication, and counselling. They can foster sustainable programming (Aggarwal 2004) via: (*a*) promoting ownership among partners of programme objectives and processes; (*b*) facilitating healthcare funding through various sources including community contributions; and (*c*) encouraging the humanistic paradigm in programming and minimising exclusion and inequity. One of the important techniques for promoting egalitarian dialogue and communication between community members and healthcare professionals for community intervention is the use of education to empower people through mediating structures, networks and community institutions (Revenson and Schiaffino 2000; Winett et al. 1989).

It is high time that NGOs maximise their efforts to promote healthcare services that are sensitive, responsive and adaptive to the diversity of the population and users' cultural and linguistic identities and their life histories. Special care should be taken to promote more equitable and effective access to healthcare services among marginalised sections of the population, particularly those who came as immigrants or refugees. A greater appreciation of the role of NGOs in the healthcare system, particularly with respect to marginalised sections of the population, in the identification of healthcare needs, cultural interpretation, access and facilitation of institutional adaptation and delivery of services, needs to be promoted. Figure 5.1 provides a model of participatory praxis in community mental healthcare.

NAMI India and Experiential Lessons

A partner of NAMI USA, NAMI India is a voluntary organisation with its head office at Mumbai. It is an advocacy and support group set up for those interested in the welfare of persons with mental problems. It operates virtually as well as physically by the contributions of active volunteers, members and branches all over India. It assists consumers and caregivers to approach the right places for treatment and rehabilitation.

In the initial stages, NAMI emerged basically as an online support group. It aimed to function as a registered trust or society, to help in the eradication and treatment of mental illness in India by integrating and involving consumers, the mentally challenged, doctors,

Figure 5.1 Model of Participatory Dialogic Praxis in Community Mental Healthcare, Its Concerns and Challenges

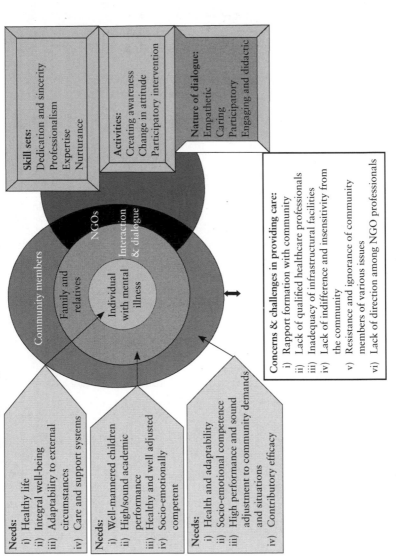

Skill sets:
Dedication and sincerity
Professionalism
Expertise
Nurturance

Activities:
Creating awareness
Change in attitude
Participatory intervention

Nature of dialogue:
Empathetic
Caring
Participatory
Engaging and didactic

Community members

NGOs

Family and relatives

Individual with mental illness

Interaction & dialogue

Concerns & challenges in providing care:
i)   Rapport formation with community
ii) Lack of qualified healthcare professionals
iii) Inadequacy of infrastructural facilities
iv) Lack of indifference and insensitivity from the community
v)   Resistance and ignorance of community members of various issues
vi) Lack of direction among NGO professionals

Needs:
i)   Healthy life
ii) Integral well-being
iii) Adaptability to external circumstances
iv) Care and support systems

Needs:
i)   Well-mannered children
ii) High/sound academic performance
iii) Healthy and well adjusted
iv) Socio-emotionally competent

Needs:
i)   Health and adaptability
ii) Socio-emotional competence
iii) High performance and sound adjustment to community demands and situations
iv) Contributory efficacy

Source: Prepared by the author.

healthcare workers, government and other sections of society. Gradually it shaped its work functions and reoriented itself with a larger focus by including the problems and concerns of people. Initially, NAMI India was formed as a consumer advocacy group for the mentally ill. However, it has now started working for the mentally handicapped, the emotionally disturbed, the hyperactive and those suffering from attention deficit disorder. The basic area of focus is the eradication and treatment of mental illness in India. M. Aniruddha (2008), a doctor, observes:

> The great thing about running Help, the world's largest patient education library, is that I meet so many interesting people. One who has especially impressed me is Akila Maheswari, who runs NAMI, which aims to dispel the myths about mental illness in India. What is really unusual about her is that she has schizophrenia — and is proud of it. Life has served her lemons — from which she has made lemonade, which she shares with the rest of the world!

The Key Objectives of NAMI

The principal objectives of NAMI include the following:

1. To eradicate the stigma associated with mental illness in our society
2. To make available treatment and medication to all sections of society
3. To be a nodal agency to support the rights of persons who are or have been treated for mental illness
4. To help in the reintegration of people with mental illness in our society

Since the beginning, NAMI India has set itself apart from other organisations with its unique insight into the problems of the mentally ill, and by taking a more pragmatic approach to the issue with a more prudent focus. The various activities of the organisation have grown more diverse and inclusive over the years, getting involved profusely with community members, organisations and key or influential stakeholders. Some of NAMI's basic activities include publicising the occurrence of mental illness in our society through various media, and educating the community against the stigma of mental illness.

Membership of NAMI India is open to all members of society, i.e., from any part of India, and perhaps the world. Initially, it was proposed that membership would be free for the first two years of NAMI's operation. However, considering the financial constraints of people in a developing country like India, membership of NAMI is still free. The organisation encourages all sections of the population to join hands for the cause of people with mental illness and those who are affected by it. It enjoys an ample amount of freedom in policy formulation, execution and implementation, and has been collaborating with several other associations in addition to opening several branches. At present, NAMI has branches in almost all the big Indian cities and is targeting small towns gradually. It has, in recent years, received assistance from eminent specialists in the field of mental healthcare in India and active community involvement.

Key Campaigns and Activities of NAMI India

Use of ICT as a Tool of Awareness and Intervention

The present age is marked by advancements in the technological sector as well as a high rate of dependence on the use of modern technologies. The exploitation of technology has seen unprecedented growth and development in almost all sections of society. The use of ICT in the healthcare sector is gaining immense popularity, especially in institutions of medical practice. However, the use of ICT in public health has not been given its due in developing countries like India. While NGOs use ICT for health, it has been observed that very few are catering to the mental health needs of the community. Innovations in this sector have been quite successful in western countries; however we do have a few NGOs who have integrated the recent developments in the ICT sector for the cause of mental health in India.

One such NGO has been NAMI, which chose to integrate ICT as a potent medium for reaching every population that has access to these techniques. It started in 2004, when major metropolitan cities like Mumbai, Kolkata, Delhi and Bengaluru were targeted as nodal centres for spreading awareness regarding its usage. The first issue was collecting the large funds required for creating infrastructural facilities, and the second was ascertaining if services could be provided from a nodal centre. As these issues surfaced, solutions had to be found. This started the involvement of qualified community members, who had access to these new media and were adept with their usage. Counsellors and key personnel were appointed in every corner of the city, as they could be a ready source of help and support in case of need. The programme involved the following five steps:

1. A software-based interactive club was started online, consisting of user groups basically catering to three sections of society who are associated with mental illness, i.e., patients (recovered and afflicted), family, and finally caregivers including psychiatrists, neurologists, paediatricians, clinical and counselling psychologists, psychiatric social workers, nurses, physiotherapists and occupational therapists drawn from several eminent hospitals and clinics of Delhi and the National Capital Region (NCR).

2. A list of professionals and their addresses has been made available online for everyone concerned, so that they can use these anytime to contact and consult regarding their concerns. A considerable amount of material has also been posted online on various diseases, simple facts about acute conditions, their aetiology, symptoms, tips for recognition problems, first-aid and emergent actions. Volunteers spread the message to their communities and publicise this intervention so that people get to know about these services.

3. An online discussion group consisting of all stakeholders posted several concerns, viewpoints, and suggestions regarding the concerns raised by group members. The most beneficial aspect of these facilities is the self-explanatory procedure for communication and posting of messages, which can be performed quite simply by any individual who is averagely literate and is acquainted with computer usage. Keeping in mind the multicultural entity of India, the website also consists of a translation facility and scripts for writing and communicating in other Indian languages.

4. Individuals can also communicate with each other online using the chat-room facility by sending instant messages, or holding conferences regarding the concerns of any one group in a multi-user environment. This has created a systemic modality for dialogue and communication and increased support and empathetic reflection from different user groups towards patients and caregivers.

5. Use of telemedicine is a recent advancement of NAMI's attempt to come closer to the community and lay the ground for increasing mass participation in the cause and generate rich dialogue inspiring the formation of new models.

Recently, the new technology of videoconferencing has been adopted in collaboration with Dr Ram Manohar Lohia Hospital. This facility, which is available in the hospital, is being harnessed to leverage the expertise of the professionals of the centre. With active help being provided by the head of the Department of Psychiatry, there have been collaborations with other NGOs in the NCR and in north India, especially in Lucknow, Kanpur and Haryana. These NGOs assemble people when they require e-conferencing to be provided (usually once in a month), and doctors from the hospital give lectures and counsel patients. Patients/caregivers from remote locations can consult doctors who can suggest new, effective medicines available for a particular disorder, describe their potential side effects, warn people about banned drugs, and so on. Recently, this technology has been used to build capacities by providing training sessions to community health workers and hospital staff in other remote locations.

E-healthcare services are being provided on the NAMI India website, which updates lists of professionals and experts from all corners of India who are on the NAMI board or are involved as resource personnel. The website also offers links to several NGOs and voluntary organisations working on similar fronts and in other related areas in India as well as abroad. It provides a customised chat-room which acts as a forum for discussion of issues among patients and caregivers assisted by trained psychologists and counsellors, as well as offering a social networking opportunity. The local involvement of the community in preparing culturally acceptable materials for sexual and reproductive health issues is important. This potential can be realised by leveraging networking and e-based healthcare services to cover the vast subcontinent of India.

Free Helpline for Mental Health Promotion

Initiated as an experiment, the NAMI helpline is now a full-fledged operation, with more than 300 counsellors available online, anytime. The organisation boasts of the use of telecommuting practices by its personnel, as they can render their services from any corner of the world, since they are always attached to internet services and can respond to the concerns and questions of patients and their caregivers. Several voluntary organisations are contributing towards spreading awareness regarding mental illness. This public awareness, and emphasis on the fact that most brain disorders are 'treatable' if diagnosed at an early stage, have a significant role to play in our health-deprived country. Help may be sought if tension, stress, fear or worry cause disturbed sleep, emotional problems, loss of interest in studies, obstinacy, irritability, a non-cooperative attitude, social withdrawal, lack of concentration, or any other problem in any individual. It was with the far-sighted agenda of spreading awareness and providing immediate help to the mentally ill and their caregivers that a helpline was initiated in 2005 in Mumbai, Delhi and Bengaluru. Notices regarding this free helpline service were dispatched to several schools and colleges in Delhi and its NCR, so that students and others could avail of this service. The helpline was planned to operate round the clock. The generous assistance/sponsorship of a pharmaceutical company helped in providing honorariums to the counsellors and experts involved in providing the helpline services.

NAMI India: Starting a Group for Obsessive Compulsive Disorder

A group for obsessive compulsive disorder has been begun by NAMI India. All those who want to join and be a part of this group are welcome. Confidentiality is maintained for those who do not want to disclose their identity. The meeting takes place every second Saturday of the month at 2.30 p.m. at the Health Education Library for People near Chhatrapati Shivaji Terminus, Mumbai. Active participation is required, as this activity is in its initial phase with regard to the formation of the group, the working of the group, the expectations from group activity, etc.

Film Production and Showcasing by NAMI India

Several videos with a deep focus on the rich Indian culture have been produced by NAMI India. These are in the regional languages, and will be aired on different channels. The appeal reads: 'We need you. All people and families of loved ones, suffering from mental illness in India, need this platform'. The specific objectives are to provide:

1. education for families, the community and mental health professionals
2. advocacy, by keeping issues related to mental illness in the public eye
3. support systems for family members of people with a neurological brain disorder
4. supporting institutions conducting research into neurological brain disorders
5. dissemination of information and referrals for people seeking help
6. information about breakthroughs in antipsychotic medication

In addition, NAMI has been instrumental in organising and winning the Genesis Film Project by showcasing the concerns of the mentally ill. Filmmakers have captured the organisation's mission, its achievements, difficulties, and the heart of the people who make the organisation work. The primary goal of this project was to initiate a forum through the medium of stories — to strike a chord within oneself and with other filmmakers to inspire and make films that matter. It also gives NAMI an opportunity to connect with local charities that are dedicated to the uplift of others. These short videos could later be used to create awareness. A film show was organised on 12 October 2005 in Dr Ram Manohar Lohia Hospital, New Delhi, on the theme of mental illness.

Involvement of Specialists and Community Interaction

Eminent experts in the field of mental healthcare like Dr Chittaranjan Andrade (psychological medicine) at the National Institute of Mental Health and Neurosciences (NIMHANS), Bengaluru, Dr Smitha Deshpande (Dr Ram Manohar Lohia Hospital, New Delhi), and others have joined the league of NAMI India and are regular consultants for its projects. They also provide suggestions to patients and caregivers.

Collaboration with Other Organisations

Cultural stigma, discrimination, and a fragmented mental health system continue to entrap people with mental illnesses in lives of quiet desperation, and endanger their lives. In response to these problems, in July 2006, A Source of Hope for All (ASHA) International launched its signature programme, the *'Rally for Recovery World Tour'*.[3] It was the first of its kind, a global public education campaign led by individuals living with mental illness. Rally for Recovery seeks to improve the general understanding of mental illness and promotes recovery. With grassroots support from mental health and community organisations around the world, Rally for Recovery accomplishes its goals through rallies held across the world. The goal of these rallies is to develop collaborative partnerships with mental health organisations around the world and to hold the Rally for Recovery event annually. Partners are offered a menu of programmes to choose from, and the programmes are customised to best serve the needs of audiences. Some of the famous programmes have been: 'A Candle in the Dark: A Journey from Adversity to Advocacy'; 'Real People, Real Recovery'; 'Demystifying Mental Illness', a community education programme that educates, empowers and inspires audiences to join forces in paving the path to recovery; 'THRIVE: Transforming Trauma into Triumph — A Recovery Institute', and many others.

Assistance was provided by NAMI India to ASHA in telecasting the programme *Out of the Shadow* (winner of the prestigious 2006 NAMI Media Award). The film festival and workshops have included other documentary films like *Men Get Depression* and *Documenting Our Presence: Multicultural Experiences of Mental Illness*. These activities were conducted with the specific purpose of engaging and empowering the four pillars of recovery — individuals with mental illness, their families, care providers and communities, to create a person-centred, culturally competent, recovery-oriented system of care. Therefore, the targeted audience included individuals with mental health problems, their families and care providers, healthcare providers and students in the allied medical and healthcare fields, the general public, community leaders, educators, employers, business leaders, human resources professionals, policy makers, religious/spiritual leaders, civic organisations, law enforcement officers, the media, etc.

The basic learning goals with which these programmes engage all the key stakeholders in the process of workshops are:

1. *Information*: to educate audiences about the epidemiology, incidence and impact of mental illness

2. *Inspiration*: to inspire audiences with a resounding message of hope and recovery; and
3. *Transformation*: to provide audiences with practical tips and tools to transform mental healthcare.

Collaboration with the Community Outreach Centre at Dr Ram Manohar Lohia Hospital

The community outreach centre is one of the attractive features of the Dr Ram Manohar Lohia Hospital, as no other hospital in Delhi provides such a formal establishment of services to the people. This centre is equipped with a TV, projector and blackboard for demonstrations and other events. The community centre has a seating capacity of 60, and consists of an airy room equipped with good ventilation, water cooler, and other facilities. It is adorned with the pictures and posters developed by occupational therapists, as most of the services of this speciality are provided in this room. Every Saturday, the centre organises some kind of public awareness programme like alcoholics anonymous, group therapies for patients and their caregivers, motivating talks (e.g., 'Yoga for Mental Health' by Dr S. N. Pandey), among other events. The activities of the whole year will be discussed later in greater detail.

NAMI Walks 2006

World Mental Health Day was celebrated by NAMI India on 8 October 2006, in collaboration with Dr Ram Manohar Lohia Hospital, New Delhi, and a few other NGOs and voluntary organisations, by organising a walk. The basic objective of the peaceful walk was to inform, spread awareness and empower people to stand up against stigma and discrimination towards persons with mental illnesses. The key agenda was to spread awareness regarding the various stagnant laws and statutes of India — the Disability Act, National Trust Act, and the Rehabilitation Council of India Act. The walk was also intended to promote mental health awareness and raise funds for continuing research. A group of over 800 people walked on Sunday afternoon from Ram Manohar Lohia Hospital to India Gate, where a congregation of eminent public healthcare specialists including psychiatrists, clinical and counselling psychologists, physiotherapists, occupational therapists and health administrators from various agencies talked on issues in mental healthcare in India.

The most gratifying of all was NAMI's instrumental role in facilitating nearly 800 walkers — people with mental illness and their loved ones — to emerge triumphantly out of the dark and into the light of a new era wherein people with mental illness would be treated with compassion and not condemnation. In Bengaluru, NAMI India has organised a walkathon starting from the Lal Bagh main gate to the NIMHANS hospital lawns. A few of the notable successes of the walk included the exchange of information between professionals and the public; the proposal to establish NIMHANS-like institutions in all states; setting up recognised psychosocial rehabilitation centres as non/commercial establishments; the creation of job reservation for the psychosocially disabled as per the Persons with Disabilities (Equal Opportunities, Protection of Rights and Full Participation) Act, 1995; and the removal of stigma through the silver ribbon campaign.

Public Lectures/Workshops for Community Members (Focus on Patients and Caregivers)

As part of the community outreach programmes, several public lectures were organised. Some lectures in the series were on 'Rightful Living', 'Mental Aerobics', 'Stress Interventions in Everyday Life', 'The Role of Youth for Mental Health', 'From Darkness to Light: Let's Fight Together', and 'How to Take Care of Mentally Ill Patients' (for caregivers and professionals). Over the years, more than 150 such user-driven lectures, especially tailor-made for patients and caregivers, have been conducted. These are designed and oriented towards positive enablement in the lives of patients and caregivers, with a strong preventive and promotive focus in the areas of integral well-being of patients. From the interactions and the opportunities for a freewheeling voicing of their concerns, community members have given valuable suggestions, which have not only helped in energising NAMI's efforts but have also enriched its work, defined its objectives, reshaped its efforts, and facilitated collaboration in getting a clearer vision with regard to community interactions and spreading awareness regarding mental illness and care. When patients and caregivers participated in these kinds of activities, they felt included, respected and cared for, which brought back to them their lost sense of self-dignity.

Patient–Caregiver–Community Member Meetings and Community Consultations

The cause of the mentally ill and their caregivers has been championed consistently by NAMI India. The biggest advantage of its patient–caregiver meetings, which are organised twice a month at Dr Ram Manohar Lohia Hospital, is the amount of curiosity the meetings have created by the regular clients and their energetic participation. The audience, without fail, leaves the presentation with a renewed understanding of mental illness. The programme has been highly effective in addressing and dismantling the insidious chain of stigma that continues to bind the lives of people with mental illness. One of the most important achievements in this process is the increased partnership between professionals and lay persons. Partnership between professionals and people in generating health information through participatory planning is crucial for increased community participation. The involvement of people in generating information leads to the ownership and utilisation of the knowledge that has been generated (Rifkin and Pridmore 2001), and hence a greater degree of accountability and eagerness to share the same knowledge among community members.

Another important role of these meetings and public lectures is to inform, educate and thereby empower the individual and the family. The greatest asset in mobilising people for health programmes may be the people themselves. For instance, if a student is informed and educated on the strengths of community participation, he/she can be further motivated to spread the message to his/her family members and neighbours. This creates the potential of involving the illiterate poor in the rural areas of the developing world. Moreover, an informed and empowered individual within a family can be a caregiver for all the members (Bhuyan 2004) and is accountable enough to bear these responsibilities. The degree of participation can be gauged from the number and varieties of participants from all walks of life (both professionals and non-professionals) who have joined the discussion groups, discussed, fought, and contributed immensely in enriching our insight into the whole issue. This has greatly accentuated the emphasis on value-centric interventions and activities by giving an impetus to such interventions. Patients, and especially their caregivers, have pointed out the pitfalls in our system over the years, and simultaneously made us strong enough to fight for the cause with their unflinching support.

Sharing Personal Experiences and Concerns, Seeking Solutions from the Community

In a recent interview with Akila Maheswari, Gayathri Ramaprasad observes, 'I applaud Akila and her visionary team at NAMI India for their tireless efforts to empower "Beautiful Minds" in India.' In the interview, she reports the deep revelations of a painful story as well as the rise and realisation of the self and its value by the pioneer of a mental healthcare movement in India. Her personal experiences have proved to be a source of inspiration for many people suffering from mental illness and for their parents. It is worth reproducing here some excerpts from the interview which reveal her struggle and journey from a wretched, mentally ill person in the eyes of society to a person of great inspiration:

> Embraced within the protective environment of a psychiatric ward, I at last found acceptance as a human being with a disease, not a demonic delinquent who was merely 'Acting Out'! For the first time in many years, I wasn't alone in my darkness. I found many kindred spirits combating their own struggles through darkness. In their courage, I found mine, in their comfort, I found communion. The hospital staff was further instrumental in strengthening my new found acceptance. There, amidst the hospital walls, I found empowerment through education, advancement through advocacy, and sustenance through support. In essence, I learned then, and continue to live my life each day, with the courage to accept that mental illness is an illness like any other. Regardless of society's misperceptions, stigma, and the institutionalised discrimination against people living with mental illness, I accept my responsibility to live life to its fullest. I find renewed courage to change the things I can through my work as a mental health advocate, and each day, I live with the wisdom knowing the difference between things I can change, and those that I cannot. Human beings need nurturing and sustainable relationships to survive and thrive in life, just as much as they need food, water, and shelter.

Gayathri Ramaprasad shares her story of how she discovered meaning in her life out of the painful and dehumanising days in the isolation cell where she was secluded under lock and key. She says it instilled in her a rage that could only be quenched by reclaiming her equity, dignity and humanity, even if required her to travel a road less travelled, alone and in terror. She continues:

> For every moment that I was forced to live in the dark indignity of depression, for every tear that I ever shed in desperate need for understanding and compassion, I found the motivation in my epiphany 'Breakdowns are Opportunities for Breakthroughs'. Entombed amidst the deathly silence of the isolation cell, I found my calling to be 'A Candle in the Dark'! Inspired by the courageous struggles of my brethren within the psychiatric ward, I discovered my true purpose in life to 'Engender a world of equity, dignity, and humanity for all individuals living with mental illness'. In my state of utter brokenness, I broke through to realise my mission to 'Empower Beautiful Minds around the World'.

Community Outreach Programmes

Counselling and online help are not the only activities of NAMI India. During 2006, NAMI initially decided to explore and venture into the communities in Delhi, basically low-income or middle-income groups. Gradually, the need to serve the needs and concerns of the disadvantaged population became more apparent. In the beginning, these ideas came out of a series of discussions with experts and professionals, which were enriched by the inputs of regular patients and caregivers visiting the facilities at Dr Ram Manohar Lohia Hospital. This made NAMI realise the importance of such explorations. The first aim was the identification of children and adolescent groups who are very vulnerable to several forms of socio-emotional and behavioural signs and symptoms which had hitherto gone unrecognised by all. In an economically weak country like ours, early signs of illness are rarely recognised until they develop into full-blown syndromal characteristics. The reasons behind this lack of recognition are manifold — basically, the lack of awareness and a preoccupation with fulfilling the incessant, basic needs of life.

The first goal was screening children and adolescents who were exhibiting, or likely to exhibit or develop, any symptoms of mental disorders after a certain period of time. We developed a set of screening tools in consultation with specialists from Dr Ram Manohar Lohia Hospital, the Vidyasagar Institute of Mental Health and Neuro-Sciences, and some experts from Delhi University and the

All India Institute of Medical Sciences. These tools were used as screening tools (which were made available in Hindi and English) in addition to the standardised psychological batteries like the childhood psychology measurement schedule developed by Malavika Kapur, NIMHANS. For spreading awareness regarding the use of these tools and the need for such screening, we sent the toolkit to almost 175 schools (both public and government-run) in Delhi and the NCR. Teachers' help was sought, as they are well qualified and with a few training sessions were expected to assist us in the collection of data. Fortunately, with a degree of struggle, repeated visits and requests made to the schools, we were successful in drawing the attention of school authorities and parents.

Initially, this Herculean task of visiting schools in all parts of Delhi, rapport formation, and the task of convincing and showing the objective/rationale behind such an exercise, had seemed to be almost a figment of our imagination. Therefore, we recruited 12 interns (with background training in clinical psychology, counselling psychology, social work and nursing), who volunteered for the collection of epidemiological data by conducting the screening in schools with the help and assistance provided by schoolteachers under the guidance of the researcher and Dr Azad (a counsellor). At several stages, the process of inviting participation from schoolteachers and other authorities was complicated by the incompatibility between the time that the volunteers and school, respectively, could afford to contribute. The individuated scheduling of activities proved useful in this regard. However, the process of contact and consultation did not end with the screening; rather, it was just the first step to a larger unknown arena, which we had not attempted to tread.

The process of reaching to the public can be summarised as follows:

1. Rapport formation through creative engagement with children and administrative assistance obtained through collaborative measures and recommendations from different hospital authorities. However, it is to be noted that the process of creating an optimal group of participants was not an easy task; rather, it required a series of consistent efforts, expedited for the enablement of the recipients of care.
2. Screening of children and adolescents for identification of symptoms or signs (if any) for early prevention, which was

very well achieved by the consistent and sincere efforts of our team of young healthcare specialists. It is a matter of great satisfaction that months of our hard efforts came up with voluminous data.

3. Pre-intervention care: consistent care was taken so that children did not feel embarrassed, but rather enjoyed the whole process of psycho-diagnostics implemented on them. Some interventions like social skills training, engagement in life skills acquisition, etc., were performed that made children show their jovial and exuberant side. The biggest help came from teachers who revealed to us several unique characteristics of the children which had gone unrecognised by the interns, and a few more insights regarding how they dealt with children who had behavioural or emotional problems, the bullies, children who usually remained sad and did not participate in peer group activities because of familial problems/tensions. Their real-life experiences added value to our future interventions, which we developed in consultations with experts, and implemented at a later date with the help of teachers, as they spent more time with the children than we did. We took special care to remain present during parent–teacher meetings, as this is where we came in contact with the parents of the children we were evaluating. We talked to them about the need for a healthy mind and healthy body and the need for early identification and prevention with a series of lectures and public discussion meetings on those days. It helped us considerably as parents became conscious gradually and took great care to observe their children, and note behavioural digressions (with intensity, frequency and duration) on a daily basis, which they recorded in a journal specifically meant for recording and follow-up. These data were complemented with our records which were based on the children's diagnostic data, pre- and peri-intervention observations.

4. Analysis of data was the next step, which was itself a gigantic task requiring immediate interpretation and expertise from the interpreter. So, we collaborated with a few postgraduate students of psychology from the University of Delhi.

5. We are still in the process of working out interventions with children. The encouraging fact in the whole situation is the great inspiring contributions and participation which we have

been able to obtain from community members, which has affirmed our faith in our efforts and made us more enthusiastic. We have realised that the community can teach us several lessons that not even experts can teach, and that community participation is key to any successful intervention.

Achievements and Insights at NAMI India

Awareness regarding common drugs, both online and through counselling, was promoted in all the NAMI branches. This information was shared and spread in order to prevent the misuse of drugs due to ignorance and to save patients from suffering any side effects, e.g., modafinil.

Another achievement of NAMI India has been the emphasis placed on values-based practice (VBP) in healthcare, and spreading this awareness to practitioners as well as the public. The International Network for Philosophy and Psychiatry has written to NAMI providing 10 principles of VBP, an approach that has thus far been developed mainly in mental healthcare. With every advance in medical science and technology, however, VBP will become increasingly important in all areas of healthcare. This is because science opens up an ever wider range of choices in healthcare, and this results in better values.

The satisfying aspect is NAMI's strong focus, developed over these five years, on preventive efforts rather than just intervention. This has been partially fulfilled through our endless public meetings and discussion forums, which we have conducted in several hospitals, healthcare agencies, the University of Delhi and other educational institutions. Further, the process of dialogic relationship, which we have developed over years of perseverance with the community, has been achieved through a participatory praxis for initiating and sustaining change in the system.

Conclusion

Gayathri Ramaprasad[4] suggests that Indian 'beautiful minds' should honour themselves as human beings and reclaim their dignity, equity and humanity. She proposes the acceptance of mental illness as you would any other illness by the person suffering, while believing that recovery is a reality. A journey of a thousand miles begins with the first step — take the first step in owning your illness and claiming recovery as your goal. Mental illness, like other illnesses, develops over a prolonged period of time. It is essential to educate oneself about the symptoms, and focus on prevention and intervention, so that one does not allow it to evolve into an acute crisis. Hence, recovery will depend equally on the patient, the family and the caregiver. People should engage actively in developing strategies for a healthy, functional, successful life and find the courage to break the silence and shatter the stigma — one moment, one person, and one courageous step at a time. Only by applying and leveraging the recent developments in ICT can we reach as many people as possible with an aim to providing our services.

Only by becoming active volunteers engaged generously in this work and becoming harbingers of hope, as non-profit organisations like NAMI India and scores of others across the country are doing, can we bring about change at the microscopic, macroscopic and systemic levels. As Akila Maheswari, founder president of NAMI India, observes, 'With more affordable medication being manufactured in India, things are going to really shine for people with mental illness as we forge ahead to contribute to society and break the barriers of stigma associated with the same.'

It is to be acknowledged that stigma stems from ignorance. It is only through persistent, widespread education that one can effectively combat stigma, by systematically separating the myths from the facts. While theoretical education about mental illness as an illness holds great promise in addressing the stigma associated with such illness, experiential learning through positive, human interactions with people living with mental illness is critical to demystifying mental illness and humanising this dehumanising disorder. Although people with mental illness and their families have valid reasons to heed the power of stigma and hide the condition, it is unfortunate that we thus perpetuate the same wrongdoing that we protest. The attitude among healthcare professionals is very derogatory and questionable, and it requires an optimal amount of self-invited reflexivity regarding one's beliefs and practices. It is, therefore, essential that we find the courage to shatter the stigma, even if at a snail's pace, with gradual but progressive steps.

Notes

1. The author wishes to gratefully acknowledge the help and support provided by the authorities of NAMI India (Delhi and Mumbai), i.e., Akila Maheswari and Dr Lalita Sehgal, and all the patients and their families who enriched his insights into the field.
2. 'An Interview with Dr. Gayathri Ramaprasad', www.naamiindia.in (accessed on 1 March 2010).
3. ASHA International, 2006 Rally for Recovery, http://myasha.org/tempasha/our-work/rally-for-recovery/2006-rally-for-recovery/ (accessed on 23 January 2015).
4. 'An Interview with Dr. Gayathri Ramaprasad', www.naamiindia.in (accessed on 1 March 2010).

References

Aggarwal, S. (2004). 'Building Public Sector–NGO Partnerships for Urban RCH Services', Proceedings of the 31st Annual National Conference of the Indian Association of Preventive and Social Medicine, PGIMER, Chandigarh, 27–29 February, *Indian Journal of Community Medicine*, vol. 29, no. 5, http://www.indmedica.com/journals/pdf/iapsm/19_Building%20Public%20Sector_saggarwal.pdf (accessed on 24 January 2015).

Aniruddha, M. (2008). 'Busting myths about mental illness in India', 18 November, http://www.wellsphere.com/general-medicine-article/busting-myths-about-mental-illness-in-india/502785 (accessed on 22 January 2015).

Bhaskar, R. (1989). *The Possibility of Naturalism: A Philosophical Critique of the Contemporary Human Sciences* (2nd edn), Hemel Hempstead: Harvester.

Bhuyan, K. K. (2004). 'Health Promotion through Self-Care and Community Participation: Elements of a Proposed Programme in the Developing Countries', *BMC Public Health*, vol. 4:11.

Chatterjee, S., A. Chatterjee and S. Jain (2003). 'Developing Community-Based Services for Serious Mental Illness in a Rural Setting', in *Meeting the Mental Health Needs of Developing Countries*, edited by Vikram Patel and R. Thara, New Delhi: Sage, pp. 117–39.

Dorsey, G. N. (2010). 'Praxis: Dialogue, Reflection and Action toward a More Empowering Pedagogy', Master's thesis, San Jose State University.

Freire, P. (1970). *Pedagogy of the Oppressed*, New York: Continuum.

——— (1972a). *Pedagogy of the Oppressed*, Harmondsworth: Penguin.

——— (1972b). *Cultural Action for Freedom*, Harmondsworth: Penguin.

Kagan, C., and M. Burton (2001). 'Critical Community Psychology Praxis for the 21st Century', Paper presented to the British Psychological Society Conference, Glasgow, March, http://www.compsy.org.uk/GLASGOX5. pdf (accessed on 23 January 2015).

Kagan, C., K. Knowles, R. Lawthom and M. Burton (2000). 'Community Activism, Participation and Social Capital on a Peripheral Housing Estate', Paper presented at the European Community Psychology Conference, Bergen, September,

http://www.compsy.org.uk/bergenpaper_social_capital.pdf (accessed on 24 January 2015).

Lather, P. (1986). 'Research as Praxis', *Harvard Educational Review*, vol. 56, no. 3, pp. 247–77.

Patel, Vikram, and R. Thara (2003). *Meeting the Mental Health Needs of Developing Countries: NGO Innovations in India*, New Delhi: Sage.

Revenson, T. A., and K. M. Schiaffino (2000). 'Community-Based Health Interventions', in *Handbook of Community Psychology*, edited by Julian Rappaport and Edward Seidman, New York: Kluwer, pp. 471–93.

Rifkin, S. B., and P. Pridmore (2001). *Partners in Planning: Information, Participation and Empowerment*, London: TALC Macmillan Education Limited.

Seidman, Edward (1986). 'Justice, Values and Social Science: Unexamined Premises', in *Redefining Social Problems*, edited by Edward Seidman and Julian Rappaport, New York: Plenum Press, pp. 235–58.

WHO (World Health Organization) (1991). *Community Involvement in Health Development: Challenging Health Services*. Geneva: WHO.

6

R: An Open-Source Alternative for Statistical Research in Public Health

Raghu K. Mittal

◻

The public health researcher essentially needs statistical tools for doing research. Analysis of data can be done by various proprietary software tools like SPSS, Stata and SAS, but these tools come at a huge cost. Nowadays, various quality open-source tools for statistics are available which are free for anyone to use. In this chapter, I explore the usage of such an open-source statistical language called R, and its viability as an alternative to proprietary software for research in public health.[1]

The role of statistics in public health and preventive medicine is quite clear. It is widely used for various estimations and tests of hypotheses, and helps in making decisions to prevent widespread diseases. Since statistics is hugely important for the public health researcher, he or she faces a considerable dilemma in choosing the appropriate software to complement his or her work, as there are many software tools available in the market for general-purpose statistical calculations. Some of the tools that have achieved widespread acceptance include SPSS, Stata and SAS. All of these are excellent tools, and can cater to most of the statistical requirements a health researcher would have. However, these tools are very expensive, and hence beyond the means of various users, especially in developing countries where there is always a shortage of funds to spend on technology. So, either organisations end up spending a lot of their budgets on acquiring expensive software, or people pirate software for their use, which is an illegal practice.

In this situation, the concept of open-source has come to the rescue of researchers. Though the open-source software (OSS) movement is not new, lately it has become hugely popular, since there are large numbers of good-quality open-source alternatives available for various applications such as photo-editing, word processing, engineering drawing, simulations, and others.

Open-Source Software

Open-source software is software made available in both source code and binary form, under a licence which allows users to freely use, modify and redistribute the software without the need to pay royalties to the original software author.

Two obvious questions that arise are: why anyone would want to release their software code, and why others would want to add new utilities and functionality to someone else's software (Dudoit et al. 2003). Aside from the obvious benefits of creating a community resource that can advance the field, there are several advantages to an open-source approach to software development in a scientific environment, including:

1. Full access to the algorithms and their implementation, which allows users to understand what they are doing when they run a particular analysis
2. The ability to fix bugs and extend and improve the supplied software
3. The encouragement of good scientific computing and statistical practice by providing appropriate tools, instruction and documentation
4. The availability of a workbench of tools that allows researchers to explore and expand the methods used to analyse biological data
5. Ensuring that the international scientific community is the owner of the software tools needed to carry out research
6. Promotion of reproducible research by providing open and accessible tools with which to carry out that research (reproducible research as distinct from independent verification)

Butler et al. (2004) talk about the success of pKADS, an open-source, desktop-based knowledge management system, whose purpose is to promote knowledge sharing in government and non-government organisations. Open-source software lends itself to creating an information and communications technology (ICT) platform that provides increased ownership and local autonomy (Dravis 2003), and can be useful for developing countries like India to benefit from.

Even though the benefits of OSS are plenty, it is not very popular in India, both in terms of usage as well as in terms of contribution towards its development. This may be attributed to two major reasons:

1. People are simply not aware of all the OSS that is available today, which can replace existing proprietary software.
2. Even when they know about OSS, they are averse to using something alien and want to stick to safer and more time-tested alternatives.

It is always good to know all the alternatives available, even if people are unwilling to use open source. The option to switch to open source should always be available and known. Appropriate education to people regarding the advantages of OSS should be imparted.

Introduction to R

The name 'R' refers to the computational environment initially created by Ross Ihaka and Robert Gentleman, similar in nature to the 'S' statistical environment developed at Bell Laboratories.[2] R is OSS released under the GNU General Public License, and it has been developed and maintained by a strong team of core developers (the R-core development team), who are renowned researchers in computational disciplines. R has gained wide acceptance as a reliable and powerful computational language for statistical computing and visualisation, and is now used in many areas of scientific computation.

Requirements of the Statistical Software Package

Zhu and Kuljaca (2005) list the minimum requirements that a statistical package should fulfil for low-cost statistical teaching and analysis. These requirements can be taken as the acid test for any statistical software, thus proving that it is good enough to be used by a wide number of people. The requirements are:

1. The package should be free: R is open source and thus is free for anyone to use.
2. Ease of use: R is basically a command-line-driven statistical language, and thus it is challenging for new users to learn, but R also has a package called R-commander (Fox 2005), which is a graphical user interface (GUI) that is very similar to SPSS, and it can do all sorts of analysis that is supported by SPSS. R also has data-importing capabilities from SPSS, SAS, Stata, Minitab, etc. (R Development Core Team 2009a), and data import from databases.
3. Tutorial and teaching components of the software: R has enough documentation for teaching and tutorial use and it is a powerful environment for teaching many aspects of computational biology, including functional genomics, computational neuroscience, dynamical systems, statistical genetics and network biology (Eglen 2009).
4. Support for a certain number of statistical functions and procedures: R has support for linear regression, univariate and multivariate analysis, box-plots, normal, Chi-square and t distribution generation, scatter plots and histograms, frequency tables and Analysis of Variance (ANOVA) analysis (R Development Core Team 2009b).
5. Ability to run under Windows operating systems: R can run under Windows, Linux, Mac OS X, Unix and BSD.

Damico (2009) outlines complex survey data analysis techniques in R, with side-by-side comparisons to SAS, Stata and SUDAAN statistical software packages, thus proving that R is capable of doing the analysis performed by other proprietary statistical tools.

Modifiability and Extensibility

Open-source software is essentially modifiable with the source code available to the community. The freedom to edit code can best be described by the saying, 'think of free as in free speech, not as in free beer'. This implies that open source gives the freedom to do anything with the software at hand. This concept is central to the collaborative nature of R, where many people are working together, formally or informally.

R is also extensible in nature because of its software architecture. It is possible for R to be used as a back-end server with a custom-made GUI, thus having a completely different look and feel to it. The concept of packages is a very important aspect of extensibility in R. R has two parts, the core R software and a package system. The package system basically is for users to create or extend R using a sort of plug-ins called packages. The packaging system means that code provided by others and computing results can be shared as effective modules. The mechanism benefits from some essential tools provided in R to create, develop, test and distribute packages. R has a particular listing on its official website called the Comprehensive R Archive Network (CRAN),[3] which maintains all the packages built by various users, most of them open source as well.

There are various R packages that are now being used. Machine Learning using R (Tarca et al. 2007), the bioconductor project (Dudoit et al. 2003), and Rattle — a data-mining package for R (Williams 2009) — are some of the examples of packages that are successfully being used today among the scientific community.

Reproducible Research

The idea of reproducible research is quite simple: its aim is to provide not only a brief description (e.g., how some data has been analysed), but also to provide the code and data to allow someone else to recreate exactly the same sequence of steps (Schwab et al. 2000). R provides infrastructure for this in the form of Sweave documents. Sweave documents contain R code surrounded by documentation written in either LaTeX, HTML or OpenOffice Writer (Leisch 2002). The document is processed to extract and run the R code; output (either textual or graphical) is then inserted back into the document which is then typeset.

R also supports R-scripts, which basically consist of the commands run to do a particular analysis. R-scripts can also be used for documentation or recording purposes as the steps needed to reproduce a result.

Though writing Sweave documents takes much longer than writing R-scripts, it leads to self-documenting work that is likely to be understandable by many researchers long after it has been written, and hence is a preferred form of documentation.

Future of R

Since R is open source, and will be open source in the future, this means that future upgrades will also be free. This translates into peace of mind and no need to spend funds later on for maintenance and buying future upgrades, an attractive proposition for a developing country like India. Looking for quality OSS to extend the system should continue to be a favoured strategy for R development, as Chambers (2009) points out.

Conclusion

Statistics is inherently needed for making decisions, conducting research, verifying hypotheses and ultimately influencing administrative decisions for the public good.[4] Nowadays, OSS is bridging the digital divide by bringing the capability of the latest technology in statistics to all people. People who are incapable of affording expensive statistical tools are also benefiting from open-source research tools, thus giving impetus to good research, better decision making, disease detection, and so on.

R has become the statistical computing tool of the new age, with big companies like Google and Pfizer also using it for statistics in a big way. It is also increasingly being used by various research institutions. Thus, it is felt that the use of R for statistics is going to be beneficial for developing countries like India in the long run. Hence, its widespread use should be promoted among industry and academia alike.

—

Notes

1. Further details about R may be accessed from the following web pages:

   • 'The R Project for Statistical Computing', http://www.r-project.org/ (the main R-project website)

- 'CRAN Mirrors', http://cran.r-project.org/mirrors.html (Comprehensive R Archive Network [CRAN] mirror website)
- 'The R Manuals', http://cran.r-project.org/manuals.html (for access to various R manuals)
- *The R Journal*, http://journal.r-project.org/ (for access to *The R Journal*, the refereed journal of the R project for statistical computing)
- 'Books related to R', http://www.r-project.org/doc/bib/R-books.html; 'R Documentation', http://www.r-project.org/other-docs.html (for other documents and literature pertaining to R)

2. 'What Is R?' http://www.r-project.org/about.html (accessed on 26 January 2015).
3. 'CRAN Mirrors', http://cran.r-project.org/mirrors.html (accessed on 26 January 2015).
4. For the interested reader who wishes to explore biostatistics further, an excellent introduction to biostatistics and research methods is provided in Rao and Richard (2005).

References

Butler, T., J. Feller, A. Pope, P. Barry and C. Murphy (2004). 'Promoting Knowledge Sharing in Government and Non-Government Organisations Using Open Source Software: The pKADS Story', *Electronic Journal of e-Government*, vol. 2, no. 2, pp. 81–94.

Chambers, J. M. (2009). 'Facets of R', Special invited paper on 'The Future of R', *The R Journal*, vol. 1, no. 1, pp. 5–8.

Damico, A. (2009). 'Transitioning to R: Replicating SAS, Stata, and SUDAAN Analysis Techniques in Health Policy Data', *The R Journal*, vol. 1, no. 2, pp. 37–44.

Dravis, P. (2003). 'Open Source Software: Perspectives for Development', *info*Dev, http://www.infodev.org/infodev-files/resource/Infodev Documents_21.pdf (accessed on 26 February 2010).

Dudoit, S., R. C. Gentleman and J. Quackenbush (2003). 'Open Source Software for the Analysis of Microarray Data', *BioTechniques*, vol. 34, pp. S45–S51.

Eglen, S. J. (2009). 'A Quick Guide to Teaching R Programming to Computational Biology Students', *PLoS Computational Biology*, vol. 5, no. 8.

Fox, J. (2005). 'The R Commander: A Basic-Statistics Graphical User Interface to R', *Journal of Statistical Software*, vol. 14, no. 9.

Leisch, F. (2002). 'Sweave: Dynamic Generation of Statistical Reports Using Literate Data Analysis', in *Compstat 2002: Proceedings in*

Computational Statistics, edited by Wolfgang Härdle and Bernd Rönz, Heidelberg: Physika Verlag, pp. 575–80.

R Development Core Team (2009a). 'R Data Import/Export', http://cran.r-project.org/doc/manuals/R-data.pdf (accessed on 27 July 2009).

———— (2009b). 'An Introduction to R', http://cran.r-project.org/doc/manuals/R-intro.pdf (accessed on 27 July 2009).

Rao, P. S. S. S., and J. Richard (2005). *Introduction to Biostatistics and Research Methods* (4th edn), New Delhi: Prentice Hall.

Schwab, M., M. Karrenbach and J. Claerbout (2000). 'Making Scientific Computations Reproducible', *Computing in Science and Engineering*, vol. 2, pp. 61–67.

Tarca, A. L., V. J. Carey, X. Chen, R. Romero and S. Draghici (2007). 'Machine Learning and Its Applications to Biology', *PLoS Computational Biology*, vol. 3, no. 6.

Williams, G. J. (2009). 'Rattle: A Data Mining GUI for R', *The R Journal*, vol. 1, no. 2, pp. 45–55.

Zhu, X., and O. Kuljaca (2005). 'A Short Preview of Free Statistical Software Packages for Teaching Statistics to Industrial Technology Majors', *Journal of Industrial Technology*, vol. 21, no. 2.

7

mHealth4U

*Convergence of ICT and Mobile
Technologies for Rural Healthcare Delivery*

Repu Daman Chand, Indra Pratap Singh and Saroj Kanta Mishra

□

Advances in mobile communications and medical technologies have facilitated the development of innovative and low-cost portable tele-health tools having potential in applications for rural healthcare.[1] mHealth is the use of information and mobile communication technology to improve health systems performance. Using information and communication technologies (ICT), and especially mobile eHealth applications, is a promising way of improving user-friendliness, and possibly the overall effectiveness of self-monitoring. Mobility, as such, brings in the added value of continuous availability and timely information access. One additional benefit of ICT-based solutions is the possibility of various types of customisation, allowing support for a wider set of application requirements than was originally planned, and meeting the changing needs and targets of individuals or larger user segments.

Telemedicine is the use of medical information that is exchanged from one treatment site to another via electronic communications. The term tele-health is closely related to telemedicine. It describes remote healthcare delivery that may or may not include clinical services. Both telemedicine and tele-health may comprise videoconferencing, transmission of still medical images, document sharing and remote monitoring of vital signs. The recent evolution of wireless communication technologies has enabled telemedicine systems to operate even in the remotest places for rural health practices, hence expanding telemedicine benefits, applications and services (Pandian 2007). In developing countries like India, the majority of the people live in rural and remote locations, where even basic facilities are not available. It is very difficult to provide medical services to the doorstep in such localities. The following technical developments have taken place over and above the existing telemedicine system for delivering public health in the remotest places.

1. Computer systems: Low-cost atom-based processors were used for deploying a large number of telemedicine terminals. Current technologies like unicast/multicast work even in conditions of low bandwidth and scarce resources.

   • Desktop: a stationary computer that runs only on AC power and requires a separate monitor.
   • Notebook: a clamshell-style portable computer that can run on batteries, has a screen size larger than 10.2 inches, and/or a hard-drive capacity larger than 80GB.
   • Thin client and cloud computing: a device and/or software in a client-server network which depends primarily on a central server for processing activities, which is separate from the user terminal. Virtualisation technology has made this possible.
   • Handheld mobile tablet: a mobile computing device that can be held in the hand and does not require a surface of support for operation.

2. Communication technology: Low-cost communication facilities can now be an alternative solution for transmitting data, voice and video to nearby telemedicine-enabled service providers. With the advancement of information technology (IT), people are gradually thinking of alternative modes, like using both wired broadband, in the form of asymmetric digital subscriber line (ADSL) broadband, and wireless broadband provided by various service providers, in the form of high-speed broadband (HSB).

3. Software-based videoconferencing systems: Mobility and lower cost of devices can only be achieved by replacing hardware with software-based videoconferencing systems. Various software-based videoconferencing tools like WebEx, Homemeeting, PeopleLink, Vennfer and Vidyo conferencing systems have been used and tested at the School of

Telemedicine and Biomedical Informatics (STBMI) to evaluate the reliability of the solutions (Chand and Mishra 2009). The minimum bandwidth required for hardware-based videoconferencing is 128 kbps, but it has been found that software solutions can also work with low bandwidth.

4. Telemedicine software: Centralised telemedicine software is used to exchange medical data/information from one site to another. All medical equipment needs to be integrated with the software for capturing patient data. Software solutions have now shifted towards web-based solutions because of their portability. Hence, centralised web-based telemedicine is ideal for rural healthcare solutions.

Material and Methods

mHealth4U: Integration of ICT and Medical Equipment

mHealth4U is a mobile tele health solution designed, developed and validated by STBMI. It is available both in an aluminium polycarbonate case (airplane cabin bag size) and a standard backpack model (Figure 7.1). It consists of an atom-processor-based laptop with a Windows Vista platform and Microsoft Office, non-invasive blood pressure monitor, electrocardiogram, pulse oxymeter, spirometer, glucometer, digital thermometer, digital weighing machine and digital stethoscope. A mobile HSB data card is used to transmit data from remote areas to a tele-consultation centre. All medical equipments

Figure 7.1 mHealth4u Suitcase and Backpack Prototype Model for Rural Healthcare

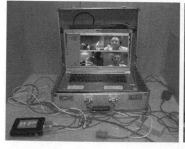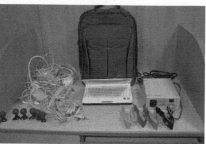

Source: Courtesy of the School of Telemedicine and Biomedical Informatics, Lucknow.

are integrated with Curesoft software. Internet Protocol (IP)–based videoconference software is used for telemedicine interactive sessions.

ICT Infrastructure

1. Computer system: mHealth4u consists of a laptop with integrated web camera, headphone and a mike. External headphones and the mike can be used for audio transmissions.
2. Communication technologies: Any IP technology can be used for transmitting the medical data as well as for videoconferencing. It is supported by any kind of internet network like Leased Line, MPLS, V-SAT, LAN, WAN and high-speed wireless broadband. Mobile phone, along with HSB, is placed inside the mHealth4u models for communication.

Medical Equipment

Both the mHealth4u backpack and suitcase models contain medical diagnostic equipments like a glucometer, digital weighing machine and vital signs monitor, which can be integrated with a laptop computer through a USB interface.

Telemedicine Software

Curesoft, a web-based telemedicine software (Figure 7.2), is used to send patient details in the form of electronic medical records (EMR) from a remote patient's end to a specialist doctor's end. The server is located in the data centre of STBMI. Remote nodes acquire the patient's data using medical diagnostic kits and Curesoft, and send it to the web server located at the data centre of STBMI. A specialist end-doctor retrieves the data from the web server after an authentication check. The entire data is stored in the MS-SQL database at the data centre at STBMI.

Web-Based Videoconferencing

The server is installed in the data centre of STBMI. Before the session, a password for the conference room is given to each of the participants. Client software needs to be installed on the computer

Figure 7.2 Screenshot of Software 'Curesoft'
Used in mHealth4U Telemedicmine Kits

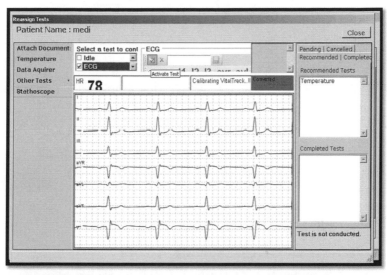

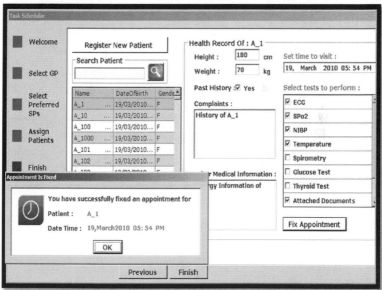

Source: Courtesy of the School of Telemedicine and Biomedical Informatics, Lucknow.

the first time. A web browser is used to open the interface web page. It has the capability of connecting to 1,000 locations, and a maximum of 40 user screens can be seen at any one time. The web interface thus gives users the flexibility of connecting from any computer.

The system was evaluated in the field. The following features were taken into account for evaluation: quality of video and audio, option of Voice over Internet Protocol (VoIP) and support of most of the industry standard protocols, installation setup, user-friendliness and machine dependency, conference recording, features of desktop and application sharing, file transfer and PowerPoint sharing, and optimum bandwidth requirement. Different types of connectivity modes, i.e., both wired and wireless based on IP, were used during the videoconference session. Currently available IP-based videoconference solutions, integrated into a low-cost telemedicine platform using both wired and wireless broadband, were included for the technical trial (Chand and Mishra 2009).

Case Study: Telemedicine-Enabled Speciality Healthcare Access for Health Emergencies

Telemedicine-enabled speciality healthcare access for health emergencies during the Jagannath Rath Yatra at Puri was initiated by STBMI, Sanjay Gandhi Post Graduate Institute of Medical Sciences, Lucknow, in collaboration with the Orissa Trust of Technical Education and Training (OTTET), Bhubaneswar. With the support of the Government of Orissa, using the technical solution designed by STBMI, OTTET provided healthcare services to a mass gathering of approximately one million people per day, from 23 June to 2 July 2009. An enterprise-based telemedicine network was set up connecting speciality hospitals at Bhubaneswar and Cuttack, using wireless broadband IP network to exchange ECG and carry out PeopleLink software–based videoconferences for tele-consultation (Singh et al. 2009).

Discussion

A telemedicine platform designed on a software-based videoconferencing system is ideal for the rural and mobile healthcare setting, and would be cost-effective over hardware-based videoconferencing solutions. Anyone can use a videoconferencing system based on internet web conferencing software to communicate with others.

There is no restriction to using a particular personal computer or location. Evolving software solutions will help further the growth, acceptance and adoption of telemedicine initiatives.

Current wireless services and infrastructure provide consumers with a variety of healthcare applications. New health IT devices and applications are made possible through wireless broadband services and infrastructure, but require additional spectrum for wireless broadband and reasonable network management. A technology-neutral approach to the universal service of rural healthcare support mechanism will help sustain the virtuous cycle of innovation and investment that has already provided many mHealth solutions. mHealth, or mobile health, involves the provision of efficient, high-quality healthcare services to mobile citizens, and u-Health or ubiquitous healthcare focuses on eHealth applications that can provide healthcare to people anywhere, at any time, using broadband and wireless mobile technologies. Keeping telemedicine costs low will enable providers to reach out to a broader audience, including those in rural areas, and to low-income patients who cannot afford to travel long distances for medical attention. Once telemedicine reaches maturity, it is not unfathomable that bringing top-notch healthcare to those who really need it will be accomplished via videoconferencing without time delay and the cost of travelling to a clinic in another state or country. Table 7.1 offers an analysis of the strengths, weaknesses, opportunities and threats (SWOT) of ICT and mobile technologies in rural healthcare delivery.

Table 7.1 SWOT Analysis of ICT and Mobile Technologies for Rural Healthcare Delivery

(S) Strength	(W) Weakness
• Low-cost telemedicine solution • Portable • Works evens with broadband connections • Less technical skill required	• Unreliable broadband mobile access in developing countries • Lack of high bandwidth connectivity like WiMAX, 3G, 4G
(O) Opportunity	(T) Threat
• Healthcare facilities at the doorstep • Healthcare system provided by an accredited social health activist • National Rural Health Mission • Equipped ambulance van	• User acceptance

Source: School of Telemedicine and Biomedical Informatics, Lucknow.

Conclusion

1. In developing countries, public health facilities should be managed jointly with telemedicine networks, for reasons of cost and efficiency.
2. Low-cost mHealth solutions like mHealth4U are the only alternative solutions for mass deployment in rural areas.
3. Healthcare based on broadband and wireless mobile technologies can reach the doorstep of people; however, technology cannot replace the physical presence of a family doctor.
4. Web and video conferencing are emerging as powerful components in telemedicine and tele-health initiatives worldwide. The integration of web-based videoconferencing has been able to help many patients, and has enabled doctors to communicate with specialists in order to make critical diagnoses faster.
5. Software solutions like PeopleLink will help to further the growth, acceptance and adoption of telemedicine initiatives.

Notes

1. The authors wish to acknowledge the Department of Information Technology, Ministry of Communication and Information Technology, and the Ministry of Health and Family Welfare, Government of India, for funding the National Resource Center project at the School of Telemedicine and Biomedical Informatics, SGPGIMS, Lucknow; and the Orissa Trust of Technical Education and Training.

References

Chand, Repu Daman, and S. K. Mishra (2009). 'Critical Evaluation of Software Based Videoconference Solution for Telemedicine', Proceedings of the HealthGIS 2009 Conference, Hyderabad, 24–26 July.

Pandian, Poondi Srinivasan (2007). 'Store and Forward Applications in Telemedicine for Wireless IP Based Networks', Journal of Network, vol. 2, no. 6, pp. 58–65.

Singh, Indra Pratap, K. N. Bhagat and S. K. Mishra (2009). 'Technical Evaluation of Low Cost Telemedicine Solution in Indian Situation: A Case Study in Ratha Yatra Festival at Puri', Proceedings of the 5th National Conference of Telemedicine Society of India, Pune, 6–8 November.

8

Using Self-Service Technology

Facilitating Customer Empowerment
in a Telemedicine Context

R. Lakshmi and P. Ganesan

■

This chapter investigates the implications of self-service technology (SST) interfaces in facilitating customer empowerment, thereby enhancing a person's involvement towards his or her healthcare. The study discusses the context of telemedicine service encounters. Based on an extensive review of existing literature, the chapter demonstrates how SST interfaces can enhance customer involvement in the pre- and post- stages of telemedicine experience. Meyer and Schwager (2007) explain customer experience as including all facets of an organisation's offering, e.g., quality of customer care, product and service features, reliability, ease of use, advertising and packaging. According to Gentile et al. (2007), a customer's experience occurs with personal involvement at different levels of rational, emotional, sensorial, physical and spiritual experiences. The present chapter seeks to contribute meaningfully by sensitising policy makers and service organisations towards an integration of available technologies to augment customer experience. Further, it also argues that there is a need for shifting from the over-emphasis on viewing telemedicine facilities in the context of the rural background, to positioning it as a service which will enhance quality medical service across the population.

Today, customers are not only worried about healthcare per se, they are also expressing a demand for greater convenience from their healthcare providers (Leopold et al. 1996). Researchers have pointed out that service providers of healthcare are waking up to the need for viewing patients as customers. The Indian health scenario needs to be understood in this context. For every 1,333 Indians, there is only one hospital bed available, and one doctor looks after the needs of 15,500 people. A huge demand for healthcare services, and a relative shortage of healthcare professionals, makes it difficult for healthcare providers to provide consistently high levels of care. In such a scenario of rapid health transition, policy makers and service providers are faced with critical issues of reforming the healthcare system. Consequently, the significance of telemedicine services as an alternative healthcare delivery system becomes very crucial.

Mair and Whitten (2000) in their study state that it is high time that research in the field of telemedicine undertook a proactive shift from the technological focus to understanding the human dimensions involved in the service encounter. There is a pressing need for realistic information that can benefit the future delivery of healthcare via telemedicine.

For the purpose of this chapter, the patient is considered as a consumer of healthcare services, and the study addresses telemedicine services from a customer-centric viewpoint. The chapter is structured in three segments. The first segment offers a review of the literature on telemedicine, customer experience, customer empowerment, SST and customer involvement. The next section discusses the proposed conceptual model along with the propositions. The concluding part talks about the implications.

Telemedicine

Darkins and Carey (2000) define telemedicine as a technology that provides an interactive, bi-directional exchange of multimedia content between a specialist and a remotely located primary care physician and patient, to facilitate the delivery of health services to the remote patient. Telemedicine has been explained by Demiris (2004) as an interaction that extends medical care service to faraway and geographically dispersed areas, persons or patients at their homes.

Telemedicine applications have been found to comprise basically two types of technology — store-and-forward technology, and two-way interactive television (IATV). In store-and-forward technology, a digital image is stored and then transmitted as part of a consultation among providers, e.g., teleradiology. The two-way IATV is used between patient and provider at one location, for a virtual face-to-face consultation with a specialist at another location. Interactive television offers the advantage of providing speciality healthcare in locations where it is otherwise not available, or in a home-care situation where it allows home-bound or isolated patients to communicate with providers without travelling to see them.

Currell et al. (2010) provide an overview of many of the latest applications of telemedicine, including remote consultations in different sub-specialities, exchange of electrocardiograms and radiological images, expert advice during emergencies in remote and harsh environments, remote foetal monitoring, and providing continuing medical education for health professionals.

The revolutionary development in the field of information technology is expected to have a decisive impact on the organisation and experience of healthcare (May et al. 2002). However, a study by Meher et al. (2009) regarding awareness among rural patients about telemedicine facilities provided by the All India Institute of Medical Sciences (AIIMS), New Delhi, found that nearly 84 per cent of the sample respondents were unaware of it. The study setting was AIIMS, and the target population included outstation patients (patients visiting the hospital for healthcare from places outside Delhi). It needs to be noted that even after 10 years of its functioning, AIIMS's Telemedicine Centre is yet to make a mark in the minds of people as a viable option of healthcare service delivery. It throws light on the fact that the involvement of both the customer and health providers is essential for acceptance of this emerging technology as a facilitator of quality healthcare service.

Customer Experience

Earlier works on experiential consumption can be traced to researchers like Holbrook and Hirschmann (1982), carried forward by Vargo and Lusch (2004) and Prahalad (2004). These researchers have worked on understanding co-creation and customer experience in their studies. Customer experience needs to be interpreted from both an information processing approach (focusing on memory-based activities), as well as processes that are 'more sub-conscious and private in nature', as discussed by Holbrook and Hirschmann (1982). This is reiterated by Schmitt (2003) and Edvardsson et al. (2005), who explain customer experience from the perspective of both normal, day-to-day actions as well as more emotional experiences. Arnold and Reynolds (2003) describe the pre-experience stage as involving the customer's anticipation and preparation for consumption by searching for information, imagining how the experience might be, and planning and budgeting for the experience.

Customers obtain value from both engaging in the experience and from the consumption, i.e., they co-create during the actual customer experience and post-experience stages (Peñaloza and Venkatesh 2006). Further, it also needs to be taken into account that in today's multi-channel environment, customers' experience in one channel may well be affected by their experiences in other channels (Konus et al. 2008; Neslin et al. 2006). In the retail context, Verhoef et al. (2009) note that customer experience involves the customer's cognitive, affective, emotional, social and physical responses to the service provider (retailer). The benefits of a positive experience are many — it enhances the customer's perceived value (Pine and Gilmore 2000) and plays a crucial role in affecting customer satisfaction, building loyalty to brands, channels and services (Badgett et al. 2007).

When we discuss customer experience in the context of telemedicine, all the three phases just discussed are meaningful — namely, pre-service experience, actual service experience and post-service experience. But the conditions or factors facilitating experience at these levels is lacking in the present situation. Can technology play a role in enhancing the experience, thereby facilitating understanding, acceptance and appreciation of telemedicine facilities among the general public?

Customer Empowerment

Wathieu et al. (2002) define consumer empowerment as letting consumers take control of variables that are conventionally predetermined by marketers. According to him, the recent advances in information technology are enabling customers to specify product or service features and prices, choose service delivery methods, control exposure to product information, and learn from other customers. Jayawardhena and Foley (2000) suggest that building customer empowerment functions in the delivery of banking services leads to cost and efficiency gains, while Hjalager (2001) proposes the empowerment of tourists as a key strategy for quality improvement in the tourism industry.

Similarly, a rising interest in customer or patient empowerment is being expressed by academics, governments and health professionals in general (Anderson 1996; Vernarec 1999). Gibson (1991) describes patient empowerment as a participatory process that would facilitate patients in identifying their own problems, and enhancing their abilities to solve these problems by identifying and acquiring the resources necessary to maintain control over their lives. Empowerment in the context of health promotion means ensuring that individuals have the necessary resources for maintaining their health and well-being (Fenne et al. 2007).

According to Bruegel (1998), patient empowerment refers to the enhanced ability of patients to actively understand and influence their own health status. Isabelle et al. (2007) point out that policies to enhance patient empowerment are mainly concerned with addressing issues related to disease management and relationships with healthcare providers.

Pires et al. (2006) opine that empowerment is a process that provides mechanisms for individuals to gain control over issues of personal concern, by developing the practical skills necessary to exert control over their decision making. According to Laschinger et al. (2010), patient empowerment happens when patients are able to access information on their health situations and find the resources and material support necessary to enable them to optimise their health outcomes. This empowerment should result in a sense of meaningfulness through self-determination and competency that helps create an impact on their lives.

Roter et al. (1988) opine that there is a greater emphasis on contributions made by patients towards medical consultations due to a paradigm shift towards preventive and patient self-care. Empowerment of customers in a healthcare context involves making thoughtful healthcare decisions, and engaging in meaningful discussions with healthcare providers, thereby influencing one's health status. An active involvement from the patient's side can improve health outcomes and reduce health costs. Lenert (2009) argues that empowered patients would be able to act in their own self-interest to make optimal decisions for their health, by being able to balance risk and benefit better.

Accessing healthcare information, especially via the internet, participation in self-help groups and malpractice claims all suggest the healthcare industry has entered an age of consumerism (Sharf 1988). A similar sentiment was expressed by Lenert (2009), that patients who had the ability to use patient-centred health information to tailor, follow up and manage treatment specific to their own unique circumstances would likely experience better continuity of care, resulting in health benefits and cost reductions associated with such self-managed healthcare.

With respect to healthcare services, MacStravic (2000) goes further by signifying that patient empowerment may benefit healthcare and managed care organisations more than consumers. This is because it potentially forces patients to make choices and take risks, and spend more time and money on treating themselves and their family members. Michie et al. (2003) argue that empowering patient–physician interactions are positively linked to health outcomes.

In the context of telemedicine, in an ideal situation, an empowered person will have the option of availing of telemedicine facilities or choosing traditional service delivery (face-to-face consultation with healthcare practitioners). The move would be made from the stage of decisions taken by the service provider (hospital/medical practitioners) to one where people will demand a telemedicine consultation. If people see encounters with telemedicine facilities as enabling them to avail of quality services conveniently, there will be a great surge in the acceptance of telemedicine services. This will definitely usher in a sea change in the way common people carry out their interactions with medical service providers.

Laschinger et al. (2010) apply Kanter's (1993) 'empowerment theory' to explain the concepts of the service provider and patient empowerment. They identify access to information, access to support, access to resources, access to opportunities to learn and grow, informal and formal power as components of patient empowering behaviours.

What role can technology play in empowering a person in the context of telemedicine service encounters?

Customer Involvement

Researchers have tried to explain involvement as determining a respondent's willingness to discriminate among dimensions. Celsi and Olson (1988) and Richins and Bloch (1986) observe that a consumer's involvement with a good service can be best explained as a function of the degree of personal relevance. Hague and Flick (1989) suggest that the higher the level of involvement, the higher will be the cognitive effort expended in the purchase, consumption and evaluation stage. Zaichkowsky (1985), Bloch and Richins (1983) and Houston and Rothschild (1978) hold that higher involvement behaviour is characterised by increased engagement in activities related to what they are involved in. Gabbott and Hogg (1999), in their study of consumer involvement in a service context, note that the degree of involvement with a product will have an influence on perceptions of service quality, while Dholakia (2001) states that involvement has an influence over subsequent customer behaviour.

Varki and Wong (2003) report that consumers having a high involvement will be more prone to having a long-term relationship with a service provider. This trend was found to be not affected by lack of choice or by the potential cost of switching. Further, customers with high involvement have higher expectations regarding their involvement in problem solving. They express a greater need to be involved with solutions to any problems that occur in the provision of the service, and are more concerned about fair treatment. When compared to products, services have been shown to be riskier due to their unique characteristics of intangibility, inseparability, etc. (Mitchell and Greatorex 1993; Murray and Schlacter 1990; Zeithaml and Bitner 1996).

Broderick and Mueller (1999) explain the product-centred, subject-centred and response-centred dimensions of involvement. While product-centred involvement entails that certain goods and services are inherently more involving, subject-centred involvement is espoused as the level of involvement felt towards a good or service by an individual. Subjective involvement has been explained as 'felt involvement' by Celsi and Olson (1988), who further add that this outlook takes into account the situational nature of involvement, as in a service encounter situation. Response-centred involvement explains the level of involvement a consumer has with outcomes related to a good or service.

Healthcare is one service that 'customers avail of with a lot of unwillingness and anxiety' (Berry et al. 2004). These are 'services customers need but may not want' (Berry and Bendapudi 2007). Moving from traditional healthcare service delivery to telemedicine facilities requires a number of attitudinal changes on the part of both service providers and the public.

Conventionally, models of involvement have been characterised based on the degree of power and level of involvement of patients and caregivers. Based on this distinction, Hanley et al. (2004) differentiate consultation, collaboration and user-controlled involvement in a hierarchy of involvement (Forbat et al. 2009). In consultations, people are asked for their opinions, which may or may not be adopted in decision making. However, they may have an influence on decision making. While collaboration is participative in nature, engaging members of the public/people who use services, the user-controlled model of involvement emphasises the dominant form of control. Here, power, initiative and ensuing decision making lie with service users. Forbat et al. (2009) identify four models of involvement which represent varying levels of participation, from consultation and collaboration to user-led initiatives. According to the authors, at the first level of involvement of user-led initiatives, consumers must be able to participate in purchasing or choosing services. At the second level of the involvement, citizens should be able to develop public policy and service plans. The third level requires involvement of all stakeholders, such as patients, service users and caretakers, in the care practice. The fourth level of involvement brings together patients, service users and their caretakers as co-researchers. Taking these factors into consideration, it is then used as justification for the proposition that if healthcare providers adopt ways to enhance consumers' involvement towards telemedicine facilities, this form of healthcare delivery will find greater acceptance among the general public.

What role can technology play in improving consumers' involvement?

Self-Service Technology

Parasuraman (2000) proposes a refined three-dimensional pyramid model, where service interactions (company, employee and customer) are mediated by technology interface. Recent technological advances have brought to the forefront the growing importance of service delivery using technology interventions (Bitner et al. 2000; Dabholkar 1996; Dabholkar and Bagozzi 2002). Self-service technologies are those technologies that facilitate customers in using a service without requiring the direct involvement of the service provider's employees.

Meuter et al. (2000) develop a classification of SSTs which divide them along two dimensions: interface (telephone/interactive voice response; online/internet; interactive kiosks; video/compact disks; and purpose (customer service, transactions, self-help). At present, most SSTs use one of these four channels: electronic kiosks, the internet, mobile devices, and the telephone (Castro et al. 2010). Healthcare kiosks, information kiosks, online and mobile-based health applications, self-help technologies, videos, compact disks, etc., are considered as various forms of SST that can be utilised in the healthcare sector.

In self-service, greater control is transferred to the customers, whereby the latter act as co-creators in the service delivery process. The role of the traditional human interaction in services is reduced or completely eliminated, and consumers need to interface and interact with technology. Recent years have seen an increase in awareness regarding SSTs, and customers have been found to be more comfortable with using these technologies. Studies by Dabholkar and Bagozzi (2002) and Meuter et al. (2000) have shown that consumers using, or planning to use, SSTs perceive them as faster, reliable, easier to use, offering greater control, and more enjoyable. Today, SSTs have a strategic role to play in the way businesses are run.

Bitner et al. (2000) point out that the conventional way of considering the customer–employee interface as a basis for marketing services has been affected by the introduction of SSTs. With the help of a technology infusion matrix framework, the authors discuss how successful application of technology can improve the service encounter. Three key drivers of service encounter dis/satisfaction suggested are: customisation/flexibility, effective service recovery, and spontaneous delight. Bitner et al. (ibid.), with the help of a critical incident study, find three major categories leading to satisfaction (helping a customer in an immediate or troubling situation, relative advantage, novelty of the technology and its ability to perform the service correctly) and four major factors leading to dissatisfaction (technology failure, process failure following the SST encounter, poor SST design, and customer-driven failure).

Objectives of This Chapter

Based on the preceding discussion of previous studies, the present chapter explores the role SST/interfaces can play in healthcare delivery through telemedicine services. To the best of the researchers' knowledge, studies concerned with the customer's viewpoint in the context of telemedicine have been overlooked, especially in the Indian context.

The following objectives are therefore considered here:

1. To examine the implications of SST/interfaces (as an information source) in empowering customers (both in the pre-telemedical experience and post-telemedical experience stages)
2. To examine the implications of customer empowerment in enhancing customer telemedicine experience
3. To explore the role played by customer experience in facilitating customers' involvement towards their healthcare

The chapter develops a conceptual model (Figure 8.1), which describes the mediating role played by SSTs in empowering customers.

Figure 8.1 SST Intervention at Various Stages of Telemedical Experience Leading to Customer Involvement

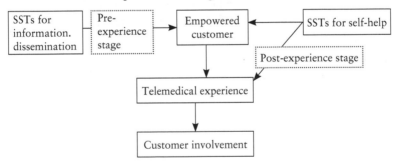

Source: Prepared by the authors.

In the context of telemedicine services, it is expected that SSTs can play a vital role in empowering the public. This role can range from providing information access about telemedicine, diseases, the rights of patients, healthcare facilities, contact information of healthcare officials, etc. (through information kiosks or SST interfaces like mobile and internet), to providing SSTs as information and experience sharing platforms. It can also enable customers to manage their health better, by providing facilities for self-care management.

Proposition 1: Engaging SST interfaces in a mediating role can empower a customer in both pre-experience and post-experience stages.

According to the health belief model (Kasl and Cobb 1966), involvement in healthcare is driven by the perceived threat of illness and the perceived benefits of and barriers to a recommended action. Roth (1994), in his qualitative study of a value-based conceptual model of healthcare involvement and preventive behaviour, discusses the dynamics of control, empowerment and trust. He suggests that the active involvement of consumers in their health and preventive behaviour enhances their confidence in being able to control their health situations and making decisions, either on their own or with the help of care providers. It builds a feeling of control, trust in the care provider, a perception of better quality of life, and peace of mind. Harris and Veinot (2004) suggest that patient empowerment enables an individual to control his or her experience of health, disease and illness through an understanding of the roles of healthcare organisations, communities and the broader healthcare system in meeting their objectives. In the context of telemedical services, a person who is empowered has clarity as to what the service can offer, which will have a significant effect on customer experience. Further, an empowered person will also make sure that any inconvenience felt during the process is discussed with the medical practitioners to find a viable solution. He or she will also act as the best promoter of telemedicine services.

The following propositions are therefore suggested:

Proposition 2: Customer empowerment will aid in enhancing a positive customer experience regarding telemedical service.

Proposition 3: Positive customer experience of telemedical service will enhance customer involvement.

Policy Implications

Globalisation is placing the social framework of a majority of nations under pressure, and the performance of health systems apparently leaves a lot to be desired. India is facing an alarming increase in changes in its disease profile, disparity between demand levels and available resources, an ever-growing population, increased medical expenses and also, slowly but surely, a generation that is demanding quality medical care. India is also an exception across countries, in that nearly four-fifths of its healthcare expenditure is out-of-pocket.

Citizens are increasingly becoming more intolerant with the malfunctioning of health service delivery systems. The need of the hour is very clear — a health system which is proactive to the challenges of a dynamic world. Verhoeven et al. (2007) argue that systems that provide an integrated environment of application tools for information dissemination, self-assessment, decision support and behaviour change have the potential to provide similar or better quality of care at reduced costs.

However, the success of any investments made in the field of technology is, to a great extent, reliant on the number of users considering technology adoption. It is also affected by the more specific attitudes towards the technological application ultimately offered. A recent study among African-Americans and the Latino population by George et al. (2009) finds a marked difference among the groups with regard to pre-experience perceptions about telemedicine. African-Americans in general expressed concerns about the physical absence of the physician specialist, the ability to monitor the specialist's qualifications with telemedicine, and the use of technology and the resulting privacy/confidentiality issues. The Latino participants were more concerned about whether telemedicine would be made accessible to the uninsured. However, both groups were equally worried about telemedical services' ability to accurately diagnose their medical condition.

Healthcare being a credence service, the relationship between doctor and patient (provider–patient) is very critical for an effective and efficient service encounter. Murray (1991) points out that service encounters high in credence qualities are characterised by uncertainty, ambiguity and lack of pre-purchase information. In the context of telemedicine services, an increased sensitivity from the side of service providers is therefore very vital. For a person used to traditional face-to-face consultation, a virtual face-to-face consultation with a specialist at another location may be met with anxiety and apprehensions about its efficacy. This is where information dissemination regarding telemedicine services becomes very crucial. Facilitating information exchange can play a major role in creating awareness as well as bringing in a positive change among the public regarding telemedicine services. It has to be understood by all the stakeholders that a very significant reason for any technology development in the healthcare field is an enhancement of the services that can be provided to the public.

Modes of empowering patients have varied from facilitating the physician–patient interaction (Little et al. 2004) to encouraging patient involvement in treatment decision making (Guro et al. 2007), as well as promoting patient self-care management programmes (Forster et al. 2007; Lorig et al. 2001). Adapting therapeutic practice from traditional face-to-face exchange to remote technology based delivery presents challenges for the service providers as well as the patient. However, patient empowerment is a significant step towards reducing the resistance towards telemedicine facilities. Healthcare service delivery using telemedicine facilities can be considered a success only when the community starts seeing it as an effective option for availing of quality and convenient medical services, and a demand for the same is created among the general public.

One of the main issues with the current management of telemedicine facilities in India is the way in which stakeholders see it as a system to reach out to people in rural or far-flung areas. Although this aspect — of healthcare reaching rural areas — is very important, confining the role of telemedicine services to addressing a particular group or a particular region limits the scope of what the service or technology entails. What is required is a system where people, irrespective of their economic background and the rural–urban divide, can make use of the system. For this, an effective network of hospitals has to be in place, and a dedicated telemedicine facility across the nation has to be made operational. Telemedicine services have to be developed as an alternative healthcare delivery option.

The present study highlights the fact that an appreciation of the convergence of technologies in improving healthcare delivery needs to be given greater impetus by both the government and healthcare providers. Meuter et al. (2000) conceptualise SST as providing customer service, transactions and self-help options. Self-service technologies can play a vital role in bringing information closer to customers (through the use of kiosks, internet, etc.) as well as in providing self-help technologies to manage self-care effectively. Arvidsson (2008) describes co-production as one of the most important, fundamental trends in contemporary consumer society. He further states that, with escalation in technology usage, this trend will be of great significance in the years to come. Greater responsibility shown by people towards their healthcare has the potential to bring in a profound change in the functioning of the healthcare sector as such.

Greater effort is needed to make technological interventions accessible to common people so that they have better control over their lives. The SST implementation should be seen as an aiding mechanism for improved service delivery by both the service provider and customer, which will go a long way towards reducing resistance to its adoption. A proper feedback mechanism planned according to the needs of the target customer base is also very crucial for its success. Further, there has to be clarity among the stakeholders regarding the type of consultations suitable for tele-consulting, as well as an understanding of its effect on consultations, its advantages and limitations (Mair and Whitten 2000).

Successful implementation and long-term usability of new technologies will require close collaboration among service providers and customers. User-friendliness, quality of care and implementation of the technology are key elements in creating an efficient and effective telemedicine service encounter. To foster widespread use of telemedicine facilities, the needs of end users should be the starting point for the development of such applications.

For such a change in the healthcare scenario, opportunities have to be created for people to know more about the telemedicine facilities as well as to share their telemedical experiences. Additionally, there should be a system in place for imbibing the feedback from the patient side, which should be taken into account for improving and enhancing the telemedicine services. Therefore, there is a need for a judicious blend of the traditional human interaction, ICT interventions and introduction of SSTs in the healthcare sector to usher in an effective and efficient service experience.

—

References

Anderson, J. M. (1996). 'Section H Empowering Patients: Issues and Strategies', *Social Science & Medicine*, vol. 43, no. 5, pp. 697–705.

Arnold, M. J., and K. E. Reynolds (2003). 'Hedonic Shopping Motivations', *Journal of Retailing*, vol. 79, no. 2, pp. 77–95.

Arvidsson, A. (2008). 'The Ethical Economy of Customer Coproduction', *Journal of Macromarketing*, vol. 4, pp. 326–38.

Badgett, Melody, Maureen Stancik Boyce and Herb Kleinberger (2007). *Turning Shoppers into Advocates*, New York: IBM Institute for Business Value.

Berry, L. L., and N. Bendapudi (2007). 'Health Care: A Fertile Field for Service Research', *Journal of Service Research*, vol. 10, pp. 111–22.

Berry, L. L., M. M. Ann and M. B. Donald (2004). 'A Health Care Agenda for Business', *Sloan Management Review*, vol. 45, Summer, pp. 56–64.

Bitner, M. J., S. W. Brown and M. L. Meuter (2000). 'Technology Infusion in Service Encounters', *Journal of the Academy of Marketing Science*, vol. 28, no. 1, pp. 138–49.

Bloch, Peter H., and Marsha L. Richins (1983). 'A Theoretical Model for the Study of Product Importance Perceptions', *Journal of Marketing*, vol. 47, Summer, pp. 69–81.

Broderick, A. J., and R. D. Mueller (1999). 'A Theoretical and Empirical Exegesis of the Consumer Involvement Construct: The Psychology of the Food Shopper', *Journal of Marketing Theory and Practice*, vol. 7, no. 4, pp. 97–108.

Bruegel, R. B. (1998). 'Patient Empowerment: A Trend That Matters', *Journal of AHIMA*, vol. 69, no. 8, pp. 30–33.

Castro, Daniel, Robert Atkinson and Stephen Ezell (2010). 'Embracing the Self-Service Economy', The Information Technology and Innovation Foundation, April.

Celsi, R., and J. C. Olson (1988). 'The Role of Involvement in Attention and Comprehension Processes', *Journal of Consumer Research*, vol. 15, pp. 210–14.

Currell, R., C. Urquhart, P. Wainwright and R. Lewis (2010). 'Telemedicine versus Face to Face Patient Care: Effects on Professional Practice and Health Care Outcomes', *Cochrane Database of Systematic Reviews*, no. 2, doi: 10.1002/14651858.CD002098.

Dabholkar, P. A. (1996). 'Consumer Evaluations of New Technology-Based Self-Service Options: An Investigation of Alternative Models of Service Quality', *International Journal of Research in Marketing*, vol. 13, no. 1, pp. 29–51.

Dabholkar, P. A., and R. P. Bagozzi (2002). 'An Attitudinal Model of Technology-Based Self-Service: Moderating Effects of Consumer Traits and Situational Factors', *Journal of the Academy of Marketing Science*, vol. 30, no. 3, pp. 184–201.

Darkins, A., and M. Carey (2000). *Telemedicine and Telehealth*, New York: Springer.

Demiris, G. (2004). 'Electronic Home Healthcare: Concepts and Challenges', *International Journal of Electronic Healthcare*, vol. 1, pp. 1, 4–16.

Dholakia, U. M. (2001). 'A Motivational Process Model of Product Involvement and Consumer Risk Perception', *European Journal of Marketing*, vol. 35, nos 11–12, pp. 1340–60.

Edvardsson, B., B. Enquist and R. Johnston (2005). 'Co-creating Customer Value through Hyper Reality in the Prepurchase Service Experience', *Journal of Service Research*, vol. 8, no. 2, pp. 149–61.

Fenne, Verhoeven, et al. (2007). 'The Contribution of Teleconsultation and Videoconferencing to Diabetes Care: A Systematic Literature Review', *Journal of Medical Internet Research*, vol. 9, no. 5: e37.

Forbat, L., G. Hubbard and N. Kearney (2009). 'Patient and Public Involvement: Models and Muddles', *Journal of Clinical Nursing*, vol. 18, pp. 2547–54.

Foster, G., S. J. C. Taylor, S. E. Eldridge, J. Ramsay and C. J. Griffiths (2007). 'Self-Management Education Programmes by Lay Leaders for People with Chronic Conditions', *Cochrane Database of Systematic Reviews*, no. 4, doi: 10.1002/14651858.CD005108.pub2.

Gabbott, M., and G. Hogg (1999). 'Consumer Involvement in Services: A Replication and Extension', *Journal of Business Research*, vol. 46, pp. 159–66.

Gentile, Chiara, Nicola Spiller and Giulano Noci (2007). 'How to Sustain the Customer Experience: An Overview of Experience Components that Co-create Value with the Customer', *European Management Journal*, vol. 25, no. 5, pp. 395–410.

George, Sheba M., Alison Hamilton and Richard Baker (2009). 'Pre-experience Perceptions about Telemedicine among African Americans and Latinos in South Central Los Angeles', *Telemedicine Journal and E-Health*, vol. 15, no. 6, pp. 525–30.

Gibson, C. H. (1991). 'A Concept Analysis of Patient Empowerment', *Journal of Advanced Nursing*, vol. 16, pp. 354–61.

Guro, Huby, Jenny Brook Holt, Thompson Andrew and Tierney Alison (2007). 'Capturing the Concealed: Interprofessional Practice and Older Patients' Participation in Decision-Making about Discharge after Acute Hospitalization', *Journal of Interprofessional Care*, vol. 21, no. 1, pp. 55–67.

Hague, R. A., and L. F. Flick (1989). 'Enduring Involvement: Conceptual and Measurement Issues', *Advances in Consumer Research*, vol. 16, pp. 690–95.

Hanley, B., J. Bradburn, M. Barnes, C. Evans, H. Goodare, M. Kelson, A. Kent, S. Oliver, S. Thomas and J. Wallcraft (2004). *Involving the Public in NHS, Public Health and Social Care Research: Briefing Notes for Researchers* (2nd edn), Hampshire: INVOLVE.

Harris, R., and T. Veinot (2004). 'The Empowerment Model and Using E-Health to Distribute Information, Vancouver, BC', *Action for Health*, Simon Fraser University and the Vancouver Coastal Health Research Institute.

Hjalager, A. M. (2001). 'Quality in Tourism through the Empowerment of Tourists', *Managing Service Quality*, vol. 11, no. 4, pp. 287–95.

Holbrook, M. B., and E. C. Hirschman (1982). 'The Experiential Aspects of Consumption: Consumer Fantasies, Feelings, and Fun', *Journal of Consumer Research*, vol. 9, no. 2, pp. 132–40.

Houston, M. J., and M. L. Rothschild (1978). 'A Paradigm for Research on Consumer Involvement', Working Paper 12-77-46, University of Wisconsin.

Isabelle, Aujoulat, William d'Hoore and Alain Deccache (2007). 'Patient Empowerment in Theory and Practice: Polysemy or Cacophony?' *Patient Education and Counselling*, vol. 66, no. 1, pp. 13–20.

Jayawardhena, C., and P. Foley (2000). 'Changes in the Banking Sector: The Case of Internet Banking in the UK', *Internet Research*, vol. 10, no. 1, pp. 19–31.

Kanter, R. M. (1993). *Men and Women of the Corporation* (2nd edn), New York: Basic Books.

Kasl, Stanislav V., and Sidney Cobb (1966). 'Health Behavior, Illness Behavior and Sick Role Behavior', *Archives of Environmental Health*, vol. 12, February, pp. 246–66.

Konus, Umut, Peter C. Verhoef, and Scott A. Neslin (2008). 'Multichannel Shopper Segments and Their Covariates', *Journal of Retailing*, vol. 84, no. 4, pp. 398–413.

Laschinger, K. S. Helather, Stephanie Gilbert, M. Lesley Smith and Kate Leslie (2010). 'Towards a Comprehensive Theory of Nurse/Patient Empowerment: Applying Kanter's Empowerment Theory to Patient Care', *Journal of Nursing Management*, vol. 18, pp. 4–13.

Lenert, Leslie (2009). 'Transforming Healthcare through Patient Empowerment', *Information Knowledge Systems Management*, vol. 8, pp. 159–75.

Leopold, N., J. Cooper and C. Clancy (1996). 'Sustained Partnership in Primary Care', *Journal of Family Practice*, vol. 42, no. 2, pp. 129–37.

Little, Paul, Martina Dorward, Greg Warner, Michael Moore, Katharine Stephens, Jane Senior and Tony Kendrick (2004). 'Randomised Controlled Trial of Effect of Leaflets to Empower Patients in Consultations in Primary Care', *BMJ*, vol. 328, no. 7437, p. 441.

Lorig, K. R., D. S. Sobel, P. L. Ritter, D. Laurent and M. Hobbs (2001). 'Effect of a Self-Management Program on Patients with Chronic Disease', *Effective Clinical Practice*, vol. 4, no. 6, pp. 256–62.

MacStravic, S. (2000). 'The downside of patient empowerment: While consumers and managed care alike applaud the trend toward empowering patients, this shift has placed new and sometimes overwhelming burdens on consumers', *Health Forum Journal*, January–February, pp. 30–31.

Mair, Frances, and Pamela Whitten (2000). 'Systematic Review of Studies of Patient Satisfaction with Telemedicine', *BMJ*, vol. 320, pp. 1517–20, doi: http://dx.doi.org/10.1136/bmj.320.7248.1517.

May, C., M. Mort and F. S. Mair (2002). 'Factors Affecting the Adoption of Telehealthcare in the United Kingdom: The Policy Context and the Problem of Evidence', *Health Informatics Journal*, vol. 7, no. 3, pp. 131–34.

Meher, S. K, B. K. Rath and T. Chaudhry (2009). 'Telemedicine — Awareness and Attitude among Rural Patients', *Ukrainian Journal of Telemedicine and Medical Telematics*, vol. 7, no. 1, pp. 15–19.

Meuter, M. L., A. L. Ostrom, R. I. Roundtree and M. J. Bitner (2000). 'Self-Service Technologies: Understanding Customer Satisfaction with Technology-Based Service Encounters', *Journal of Marketing*, vol. 64, no. 3, pp. 50–64.

Meyer, Christopher, and Andre Schwager (2007). 'Understanding Customer Experience', *Harvard Business Review*, February, pp. 117–28.

Michie, S., J. Miles and J. Weinman (2003). 'Patient-Centredness in Chronic Illness: What Is It and Does It Matter?', *Patient Education and Counseling*, vol. 51, pp. 197–206.

Mitchell, V. W., and M. Greatorex (1993). 'Risk Perception and Reduction in the Purchase of Consumer Services', *The Service Industries Journal*, vol. 13, no. 4, pp. 179–200.

Murray, K. B. (1991). 'A Test of Services Marketing Theory: Consumer Information Acquisition Activities', *Journal of Marketing*, vol. 55, no. 1, pp. 10–25.

Murray, K. B., and J. L. Schlacter (1990). 'The Impact of Services versus Goods on Consumers' Assessment of Perceived Risk and Variability', *Journal of the Academy of Marketing Science*, vol. 18, no. 1, pp. 51–65.

Neslin, Scott A., et al. (2006). 'Challenges and Opportunities in Multichannel Customer Management', *Journal of Service Research*, vol. 9, no. 2, pp. 95–112.

Parasuraman, A. (2000). 'Technology Readiness Index (TRI): A Multiple-Item Scale to Measure Readiness to Embrace New Technologies', *Journal of Service Research*, vol. 2, no. 4, pp. 307–20.

Peñaloza, Lisa, and Alladi Venkatesh (2006). 'Further Evolving the New Dominant Logic of Marketing: From Services to the Social Construction of Markets', *Marketing Theory*, vol. 6, no. 3, pp. 299–316.

Pine II, B. J., and J. H. Gilmore (2000). 'Satisfaction, Sacrifice, Surprise: Three Small Steps Create One Giant Leap into the Experience Economy', *Strategy & Leadership*, vol. 28, no. 1, pp. 18–23.

Pires, Guilherme D., John Stanton and Rita Paulo (2006). 'The Internet, Consumer Empowerment and Marketing Strategies', *European Journal of Marketing*, vol. 40, nos 9–10, pp. 936–49.

Prahalad, C. K. (2004). 'The Co-creation of Value', *Journal of Marketing*, vol. 68, no. 1, p. 23.

Richins, M. L., and P. H. Bloch (1986). 'After the New Wears Off: The Temporal Context of Product Involvement', *Journal of Consumer Research*, vol. 13, pp. 280–85.

Roter, L. D., J. A. Hall and N. R. Katz (1988). 'Patient–Physician Communication: A Descriptive Summary of the Literature', *Patient Education and Counseling*, vol. 12, pp. 99–119.

Roth, S. Martin (1994). 'Enhancing Consumer Involvement in Health Care: The Dynamics of Control, Empowerment, and Trust', *Journal of Public Policy & Marketing*, vol. 13, no. 1, pp. 115–32.

Schmitt, B. H. (2003). *Customer Experience Management: A Revolutionary Approach to Connecting with Your Customers*, Hoboken, NJ: John Wiley & Sons.

Sharf, B. F. (1988). 'Teaching Patients to Speak Up: Past and Future Trends', *Patient Education and Counseling*, vol. 11, pp. 95–108.

Vargo, S. L., and R. F. Lusch (2004). 'Evolving a New Dominant Logic for Marketing', *Journal of Marketing*, vol. 68, pp. 1–17.

Varki, S., and S. Wong (2003). 'Consumer Involvement in Relationship Marketing of Services', *Journal of Service Research*, vol. 6, no. 1, pp. 83–91.

Verhoef, Peter C., et al. (2009). 'Customer Experience Creation: Determinants, Dynamics and Management Strategies', *Journal of Retailing*, vol. 85, no. 1, pp. 31–41.

Verhoeven, M., V. Gunnarsson and S. Carcillo (2007). 'Education and Health in G7 Countries: Achieving Better Outcomes with Less Spending', International Monetary Fund Working Paper WP/07/263, International Monetary Fund.

Vernarec, E. (1999). 'Health Care Power Shifts to the People', *Business & Health*, vol. 17, pp. 8–13.

Wathieu, L., L. Benner, Z. Carmon, A. Chattopadhyay, K. Wertenbroch, A. Drolet, J. Gourville, A. V. Muthukrishnan, N. Novemsky, R. K. Ratner and G. Wu (2002). 'Consumer Control and Empowerment: A Primer', *Marketing Letters*, vol. 13, no. 3, pp. 297–305.

Zaichkowsky, J. L. (1985). 'Measuring the Involvement Construct', *Journal of Consumer Research*, vol. 12, pp. 341–92.

Zeithaml, V. A., and M. J. Bitner (1996). *Services Marketing*, New York: McGraw-Hill.

9

A Framework for Mobile-Based Electronic Data Collection in Clinical Trials

Peter Wakholi, Weiqin Chen and Jørn Klungsøyr

◼

Mobile devices are increasingly replacing paper-based routines as a primary data collection platform. In clinical trials, they provide an opportunity for replacing paper as source documents. In order to adopt mobile devices, there is a need to address issues with electronic data capture (EDC) on the mobile platform as provided by Food and Drug Administration (FDA) guidelines, as well as process monitoring and flexible collaborations provided by paper-based routines. This chapter proposes a framework for the deployment of process-aware information systems for clinical trials utilising mobile-based routines as source documents. This framework is based on the process-oriented view of electronic data collection and relevant industry standards.

Clinical trials are used to evaluate newly developed products in pharmaceutical, biotechnology and medical device companies. The advent of information technologies has enabled EDC where data is captured on paper, and then entered into an electronic system — commonly web-based (Marks 2004). The paper document, in this case, acts as a source document. A source document is a document in which data collected for a clinical trial is first recorded. The data is usually later entered in the case report form (CRF). The CRF is a paper or electronic questionnaire used in clinical trial research to collect data from each participating site. In multi-site trials, the process of capturing data on paper and entering it into the system is labour-intensive, inefficient and error-prone. Despite advances in mobile computing, there still remain many impediments to replacing paper as authentic source documents.

Marks (2004) identifies the possible reasons for over-reliance on paper-based routines instead of EDCs as including FDA guidelines, lack of mobile hardware and the attitude of investigators. Currently, many field-based activities utilise mobile devices for data collection. Many tools that use forms on mobile devices for data collection have been developed (Barton et al. 2006; Kumar and Zahn 2003; Tomlinson et al. 2009). Examples of mobile devices include mobile phones, personal digital assistants, pocket personal computers and laptops. Mobile devices provide a possible platform for data collection. The open mobile electronic vaccine trials, or OMEVAC, project aims to develop a framework for mobile data collection in clinical trials (Klungsøyr 2009). To adopt mobile devices, there is need to address FDA guidelines and current paper-based practices, which have important implications for mobile device use.

The FDA guidelines for EDC require computer-generated, time-stamped audit trails to be automatically generated by electronic systems supporting clinical trials. This documentation effort should record all applicable predicates like date, time or sequencing of events and other requirements that ensure that changes to records do not obscure previous entries. In many organisations, information systems that support coordination of work, and are able to keep such logs, are referred to as process-aware information systems (PAIS) (van Dongen et al. 2005). Techniques commonly referred to as process mining that enable the automatic discovery of process models and analysis for audit purposes have also been developed (Minseok and van der Aalst 2008; van der Aalst 2005; van der Aalst et al. 2004).

The technologies and techniques just mentioned provide a good basis to address some of the challenges in the adoption of mobile devices to replace paper as authentic source documents. However, guidelines that address the limitations of mobile devices and utilise the opportunities of PAIS while maintaining the good features of paper need to be developed in order to enable digitisation of data at source using mobile devices. Taking a process-oriented view of clinical data, this chapter addresses the problem by proposing a framework that aims to achieve FDA guidelines for EDC in a mobile environment and enable monitoring of the data collection process by field teams working in remote environments.

The rest of the chapter is organised as follows. The next section discusses the FDA guidelines and their implications for PAIS solutions. This is followed by a discussion of paper-based workflow routines in clinical trials. Subsequently, we discuss how mobile devices can be modelled on workflows in paper-based routines. Then, we move on to discuss process mining techniques and their applicability in monitoring and audits. We next propose a framework to enable mobile-based EDC, monitoring and audit. After a section summarising related work, the chapter concludes with a discussion of some further considerations.

FDA Guidelines regarding EDC

The FDA guidelines for electronic data aim to keep the accuracy, reliability, integrity, availability and authenticity of paper-based records, in order to allow for audits. The FDA issued regulations that provide criteria for acceptance by FDA for computerised systems used in clinical trials (FDA 1996, 2007). In this section, we look at some process-related issues and discuss the implications for mobile data collection.

According to FDA (2007), one of the key guidelines regarding electronic records and electronic signatures provides that adequate procedures must be in place to use secure, computer-generated audit trails that are time-stamped to independently record the date and time of all operator actions involving creation, modification or deletion of electronic records. This guideline raises a number of issues that the framework should address. The provision for 'independent record' means that all devices should be capable of tracking operator activity. The system on the device should guide the operator to be systematic in the creation, modification and deletion of records. The audit trail functionality should be built into the software and is especially important for critical computer-related processes. Because field activities take place with little supervision, a predefined process would eliminate unnecessary mistakes or problems that would result from these. Workflow systems can be used for this purpose because they enable the execution of tasks based on predefined process models (Hollingsworth 1995). Moreover, each task executed can be logged by capturing information on what has been changed, who has done it, and at what time.

The guidelines also recommend that changes to any record must be documented through audit trails so that previously recorded information is always available, when required. Such audit trail documentation must be maintained for the entire life of the electronic records and be made available for review. The creation, edition and deletion of source documents in clinical trials are critical such that computer systems are required to provide for versioning of the records in order to ensure that all changes made can be traced (FDA 2007). All these activities could be captured in an audit trail. In order to accomplish this in a mobile environment, the limited computing power of mobile devices and lack of connectivity in remote areas needs to be addressed. The trail stored by the mobile device should only temporarily be held, and should be transferred to a high-end server once connection is established.

The guidelines further recommend that all computer systems used in the generation, maintenance and archiving of electronic records must be validated to ensure accuracy, reliability and consistent independent performance, and ensure that these systems are able to discern invalid or altered records. This provision provides a challenge for the mobile environment because, in the absence of a central system controlling the clinical trial process, each system on a mobile client can be regarded as a separate system. Validation on mobile devices may not be possible because of limited computing power. This means that the central server should provide for more advanced backward validation of all the data received. Again, this can be achieved by process mining the event log. We discuss process mining at a later stage in this chapter. We suggest the validation of user activity by determining the conformance of the submitted log with some predefined rules and process models.

Paper-Based Workflow Routines

A clinical trial can be understood as a workflow process. The core activities in any clinical trial include protocol development, protocol use and implementation in the experimentation, data collection and the evaluation of the results (Jarm et al. 2007). The workflows are defined based on study protocols, which specify the duration and structure of the study and the standard guidelines which must be followed by all participants (FDA 1996). The data collection process is most difficult as it involves field studies, which could be in single or multiple sites, often in remote rural environments. One of the core documents in clinical trials for data collection is the CRF.

The CRF is a form where the investigator enters all patients' clinical and non-clinical data related to the trial. There are three types of data: non-time-dependent, time-dependent and cumulative data (Moon 2006). Non-time-dependent data is the data collected at a snapshot of time. Such data includes subject demographics and medical history. Time-dependent data is data collected repeatedly over time through multiple visits. Cumulative data is data collected over time, but not linked to a specific visit. After clinical trial data is collected on the paper forms, it has to be entered in the electronic database in order to perform computer data analysis. For this purpose, investigators usually send copies of the paper CRF to the data centre where data entry into a database is done. This paper-based routine has many disadvantages which result in erroneous data in the database and longer duration of clinical trials. There is, therefore, an increasing reliance on electronic CRF, specifically web-based systems to address these challenges and improve EDC. Mobile devices provide an opportunity for EDC in developing countries due to their portability and wide use — unlike web-based systems.

Figure 9.1 shows a visual representation of a paper-based CRF environment and the corresponding set-up in the proposed mobile environment. Field teams usually have CRFs that clearly outline the

Figure 9.1 Mobile Workflow Environment Modelled on Paper-Based Routines

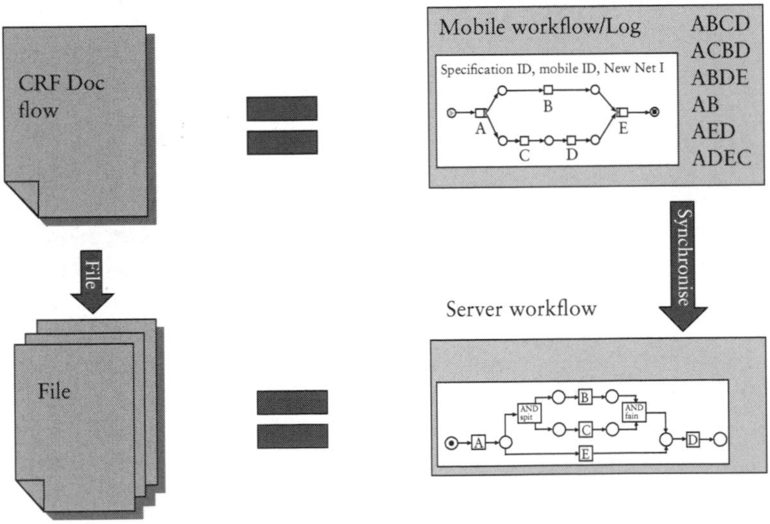

Source: Prepared by the author.

steps to be taken in the study. Forms may be those of existing cases or those used to register new cases. Once data has been captured, it is filed at a central registry. Other teams are able to access these files, evaluate the current status of work and carry out any further work. In a way, the paper-based routines therefore give a way of determining the flow of work and collaboration by enabling others to simply look through a file and continue with the process.

The workflow element of the paper-based routine is modelled using the mobile environment. The steps to be followed in the study are defined in the workflow on the server. Four possible scenarios can be used to model the paper-based routine:

1. Lone fieldworker: In this scenario, a fieldworker autonomously carries out various tasks.
2. Collaborative team: This involves a team of fieldworkers working together collaboratively to accomplish a set of tasks.
3. Centralised team: Fieldworkers carry out tasks assigned by the central office.
4. Mixed team: This scenario is a mixture of all the preceding scenarios. It represents a common environment in an organisation that seeks to use all available channels.

Mobilising Workflow Systems

Workflow Management Coalition is an international organisation that has provided a reference model to standardise how workflow management is implemented (Hollingsworth 1995). The model specifies a framework for workflow systems, identifying their characteristics, functions and interfaces. It has acted as a development standard for workflow systems. Workflows are executed based on process models which are defined at design time using constructs. These constructs include activity models, which specify activities to be undertaken; event models, which specify the current state of the process; and gateway models which define the routing. Most workflow management systems (WFMS) support workflow participants (or users) performing work activities only in office environments (Jing et al. 1999). However, the advent of mobile technologies has created opportunities for extension of these systems to field activities.

Mobile workflows are of interest because, despite the many limitations of using mobile phones, they can enable delivery of tasks directly to the mobile user's device. Because these devices are always with the user, it provides for quick response, enabling work to be executed faster. With mobile workflows, field teams are able to work collaboratively in remote areas. The elimination of paper for data collection enables instant digitisation of data, improved monitoring and reduced costs. Muller-Wilken et al. (2000) note that, 'in spite of inherent design limitations such as lack of computational power, extremely limited resources and closedness to modifications', the demand to have mobile integration to existing information systems is compelling. Bahrami et al. (2006) go on to identify the challenges of using mobile devices for field studies as relating to connectivity, security, mobility and portability. Connectivity challenges relate to the fact that a disconnection occurs when out of range. Because devices should be portable, there are limitations to resources, which results in less computational power, small display screens and storage capacity. Mobility causes the devices to use wireless communications, which are usually more costly and limited in network coverage.

Traditionally, WFMS have a process controlled by a centralised server with users performing work using remote clients. In a disconnected environment, a user would require more autonomy in starting and executing work items. Furthermore, the limitations of the mobile computing environment need to be taken into consideration in order to implement an appropriate solution. The scenarios identified previously in this section would therefore require a more flexible approach, as explained in the following:

1. Lone fieldworker (Figure 9.2, scenario 1): The user has a mobile device with a workflow engine and a workflow definition guiding the execution of tasks. The workflow engine should be able to report back to the main system on the work undertaken.
2. Collaborative team (Figure 9.2, scenario 2): In this case, one mobile device would work as a server to clients possessed by other team members. The mobile server delivers the tasks to the clients, and reports progress to the main system.
3. Centralised team (Figure 9.2, scenario 3): The main workflow engine at the central office delivers tasks to fieldworkers' mobile devices. This scenario would require the team to be constantly connected so as to receive the tasks.

Figure 9.2 Topology Diagram for Typical Application Scenario

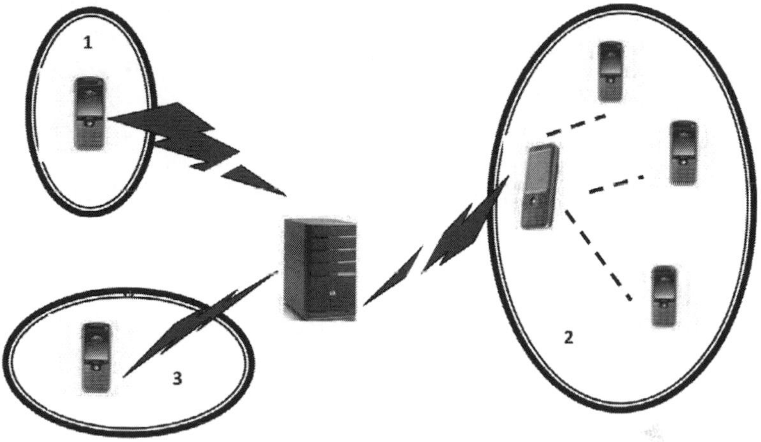

Source: Prepared by the author.

4. Mixed team: This would require distributed workflow engines collaborating to work on several tasks. Each workflow engine keeps a log of all the tasks executed. The mobile devices synchronise with a central system which coordinates all teams.

Scenarios 1, 2 and 3 need a fundamentally different approach to the architecture of many WFMSs. The architecture should provide for the definition of work to be undertaken. Based on this definition, each team autonomously proceeds to undertake tasks. An event log that notes each task and the time of execution is kept on the device. This corresponds to the paper trail of a paper-based routine. In order to keep the team up-to-date with the current work status, synchronisation is done once a connection is established. Through synchronisation, every WFMS within the distributed environment updates the Master WFMS on the tasks undertaken. The Master WFMS would then update all other systems on current status and assign new work items.

Process Awareness and Mining

Many of today's WFMS are 'process aware', in that they keep a log of all events taking place in the system. An audit trail in a clinical trial is an example of such event logs. Process mining is the extraction of non-trivial and useful information from event logs recorded by information systems. Process mining aims to discover, monitor and improve real processes (i.e., not assumed processes) by extracting knowledge from event logs (van der Aalst et al. 2004). The knowledge extracted can be used to provide feedback for auditing, analysis and improvement of business processes. Models constructed from event logs can show a representation of the process itself (ibid.). They can also be used for conformance by comparing the required process model with the event log in order to find any discrepancies. Finally, many extensions can be developed to enable new perspectives of the process, such as the control flow and organisational perspectives.

By studying the control flow discovery, it is possible to automatically construct a process model (e.g., a Petri net) describing the causal dependencies between activities (van der Aalst 2005). This can be the basis for automated audits as it would enable new insights into the process to be developed and to determine the conformance to some prescribed standards. Van der Aalst (ibid.) proposes two techniques for business process alignment — conformance testing and delta analysis. Delta analysis can be used to compare the discovered model with some predefined processes model. For example, in a clinical trial, the 'discovered model' could be the actual process undertaken, while 'predefined process model' could be a model derived from a clinical trial protocol or audit guidelines. Conformance testing can also be used to directly compare the log with the descriptive or prescriptive process model.

The organisational perspective aims at the discovery of organisational knowledge, such as organisational structures and social networks. It can be used to determine whether the right personnel worked on tasks, and to follow up any discrepancies with the concerned persons. Minseok and van der Aalst (2008) identify three kinds of organisational mining: organisational model mining, social network analysis, and information flow between organisational entities. In organisational model mining, an organisational model can be discovered from process logs. Social network analysis mines the log to discover how individuals, or groups within an organisation, interact. Using this technique, it is possible to compute metrics such as centrality, position, density, etc., that can be used for monitoring and process improvement. Information flow between organisational entities is based on social networks by showing how organisational units or roles in an organisation interact. The organisational perspective can therefore help in verifying whether the right people did the work (e.g., if a certain test was conducted by a medical doctor) — which is a key component of clinical audits. It can also be used for monitoring workloads and inefficiency in the system, hence enabling process improvement.

Proposed Framework

We envisage a scenario where users directly enter data into a mobile device so that no paper is employed or necessary. The data on a mobile device is, therefore, captured directly into a permanent electronic record. To implement such a PAIS for clinical trials, WFMS and process mining can be used to ensure conformance with the identified FDA guidelines as explained in what follows.

1. *Computer-generated, time-stamped audit trails:* There are two options to be provided here:

   a. A mobile device is equipped with a workflow definition, tasks executed follow the predefined model and a log for each task is kept.
   b. The user has a mental picture of what to do. Every task done is logged. This scenario provides for more flexibility.

2. *Keeping an audit trail:* Once the connection is established with a server, the log is submitted along with the case data. This log should be logically arranged to appear as if it were from one computer. It should also be possible to have a complete trace of the log linked with associated case data. This requires synchronisation of various collaborating systems.

3. *Validation and monitoring:* This can be undertaken at three levels:

   a. When a user submits information from a mobile device, the log is read to determine any non-conformance to a predefined model.
   b. When a complete log has been developed, some predefined audit rules can be run through the log to determine any deviations.

c. At a specific milestone of a study, the whole log can be
mined to obtain a view of the process as it is. An audit
report can then be automatically generated by visualisation
of the process.

Figure 9.3 shows a framework for utilising mobile devices for
EDC in clinical trials based on an illustration of a process mining
and information system (van der Aalst 2004). It shows the key
components (labelled 1–7) that constitute the implementation of a
process-aware workflow system capable of keeping a record of all
tasks executed. A server that has a workflow engine is used for the
enactment of workflow/process models for the clinical trial. These
models are then loaded to a mobile device which has a light-weight
workflow engine capable of supporting the clinical data collection
process and keeping an event log of the tasks specified (labels 1
and 2). The log contains information relating to the task, time of
execution, the executor and any other relevant process data. This
log serves as the basis for synchronisation and real-time monitoring
of the process. A complete log of the clinical trial consists of all the

Figure 9.3 WFMS and Process Mining to be Applied in Clinical Trials

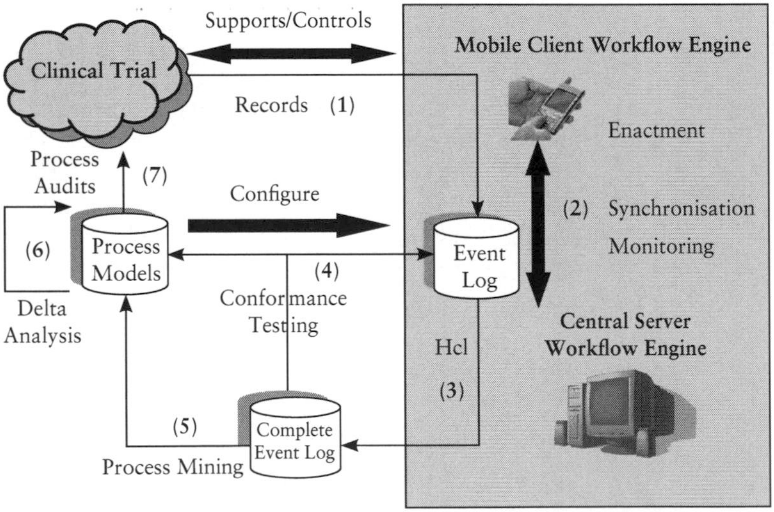

Source: Adapted from van der Aalst (2004).

logs from the data collection process on mobile devices and any other activities in the process collected over the entire clinical trial period (label 3). Conformance checking against predefined process models is conducted both on the mobile device log and the complete log (label 4). Process mining is carried out to extract a view of the actual process from the log (label 5). These models are then compared with predefined models generated from FDA guidelines and the study protocols to answer questions related to process audits (label 6 and 7).

Related Work

There are several solutions that have been developed for EDC in web-based environments. Many web-based systems utilise client-server technology that allows client software running on the investigator's computer while the server software processes data and controls the workflow (Santoro et al. 1999). An example is OpenClinica, which is an open-source tool for web-based data collection and management in clinical trials (Collins 2007). It is used to collect, manage and store data on clinical trials in an electronic database. Clinical trial systems typically keep multiple versions of documents and audit trails to maintain the integrity of source documents. This research demonstrates how process mining could be incorporated for monitoring and auditing purposes, which has not been explored by these implementations.

Mobile devices too have been used in data collection (Seebregts et al. 2008). Koop and Mösges (2002) use mobile devices in a nasal provocation study and compare the results with paper-based routines. They give a list of 'dos and don'ts' while using mobile devices in a clinical trial. They recommend that process-related guidelines be developed to emphasise the need for reminders or time-stamped data and monitoring through continuous quality improvement activities and adaptive therapies. The proposed framework addresses this, and demonstrates how this can be achieved using mobile devices. Monitoring is emphasised and the list of 'do's and don'ts' could play a role in determining what aspects of the process to monitor. Workflow systems seek to constrain user behaviour when carrying out an activity. Therefore, this research would enable the configuration of the clinical trial to ensure adherence to such guidelines.

There have been attempts to develop a framework that delivers workflow definitions to mobile devices in disconnected environments (Bahrami et al. 2006). The IBM FlowMark (Alonso et al. 1996) is an example of a meta-model that seeks to address the constraints of deploying mobile workflows. The ideas presented in the IBM model need to be extended to cater to disconnected and distributed workflows, which has been addressed in this work.

Process mining is a relatively new research area that is gaining a lot of interest. Through ProM — an extensible process mining framework, a wide variety of process mining techniques, in the form of plug-ins, have been developed (van Dongen et al. 2005). The framework has more than 230 process mining plug-ins available. They are related to control flow mining techniques, organisational perspective mining, conformance checking, verification, data visualisation and performance analysis. These techniques can be applied in a variety of situations to gain insight on processes. Being a new area, typical application scenarios of the proposed techniques need to be explored. For example, Mans et al. (2009) use process mining to discover typical paths followed by a group of patients in a hospital in order to improve care flow. The application in clinical trials provides a rich domain to illustrate how process techniques can be used to develop appropriate solutions for data collection that address the issues related to paper-based routines as described earlier in this chapter.

Conclusion and Future Work

This chapter has discussed the challenges related to the adoption of mobile devices as source documents in clinical trials. Two problems are discussed: how to retain the good attributes of paper, and how to ensure that mobile data collection follows FDA guidelines. Specific interest in process-related issues in data collection forms the basis for the proposed framework.

The proposed framework utilises workflow technologies and process mining for deployment in a mobile environment. Key issues that the framework addresses are flexibility of work in disconnected environments, tracking work progress, keeping audit trails and generating automated reports for monitoring and conformance checking.

As a proof of concept, the proposed framework will form a basis for the extension of openXdata in the OMEVAC project

(Klungsøyr 2009). The data collection tool that has been developed will be deployed along with a paper-based data collection method. Comparison of the capabilities of both methods shall then be carried out to ascertain how the proposed solution matches the existing data collection and audit practices. The system will be deployed in a clinical trial under the OMEVAC project as a case study. It will be field-tested in Africa in ongoing trials. The knowledge generated from this study will be utilised as part of the project.

—

References

Alonso, G., R. Gunthor, M. Kamath, D. Agrawal and C. Mohan (1996). 'Exotica/FMDC: A Workflow Management System for Mobile and Disconnected Clients', *Distributed and Parallel Databases*, vol. 4, no. 3, pp. 229–47.

Bahrami, A., C. Wang, J. Yuan and A. Hunt (2006). 'The Workflow Based Architecture for Mobile Information Access in Occasionally Connected Computing', Paper presented at the IEEE International Conference on Services Computing, Chicago, 18–22 September.

Barton, J., S. Zhai and S. Cousins (2006). 'Mobile Phones Will Become the Primary Personal Computing Devices', Proceedings of the Seventh IEEE Workshop on Mobile Computing Systems and Applications (WMCSA '06), doi: 10.1109/WMCSA.2006.17.

Collins, C. (2007). 'OpenClinica — Open Source for Clinical Research', http://www.openclinica.org (accessed on 5 May 2010).

FDA (Food and Drug Administration) (1996). 'Guidance for Industry, E6 Good Clinical Practice: Consolidated Guidance', http://www.fda.gov/cder/guidance/ (accessed on 28 January 2015).

——— (2007). 'Guidance for Industry Computerized Systems Used in Clinical Investigations', http://www.fda.gov/downloads/Drugs/GuidanceComplianceRegulatoryInformation/Guidances/UCM070266.pdf (accessed on 28 January 2015).

Hollingsworth, D. (1995). 'Workflow Management Coalition: The Workflow Reference Model', http://www.wfmc.org/standards/docs/tc003v11.pdf (accessed on 28 January 2015).

Jarm, T., Kramar, P. and A. Zupanic (2007). 'Reshaping Clinical Trial Data Collection Process to Use the Advantages of the Web-Based Electronic Data Collection', Paper presented at the 11th Mediterranean Conference on Medical and Biomedical Engineering and Computing, Ljubljana, Slovenia, 26–30 June.

Jing, J., K. Huff, H. Sinha, B. Hurwitz and B. Robinson (1999). 'Workflow and Application Adaptations in Mobile Environments', Proceedings of the Second IEEE Workshop on Mobile Computing Systems and Applications (WMCSA '99), New Orleans.

Klungsøyr, J. (2009). 'OMEVAC — Open Mobile Electronic Vaccine Trials', http://www.uib.no/en/rg/childhealth/67808/omevac-open-mobile-electronic-vaccine-trials (accessed on 16 February 2015).

Koop, A., and R. Mösges (2002). 'The Use of Handheld Computers in Clinical Trials', Controlled Clinical Trials, vol. 23, pp. 469–80.

Kumar, S., and C. Zahn (2003). 'Mobile Communications: Evolution and Impact on Business Operations', Technovation, vol. 23, pp. 515–20.

Mans, R. S., M. H. Schonenberg, M. Song, W. M. P. van der Aalst and P. J. M. Bakker (2009). 'Application of Process Mining in Healthcare — A Case Study in a Dutch Hospital', Biomedical Engineering Systems and Technologies, vol. 25, pp. 425–38.

Marks, R. G. (2004). 'Validating Electronic Source Data in Clinical Trials', Controlled Clinical Trials, vol. 25, pp. 437–46.

Minseok, S., and W. M. P. van der Aalst (2008). 'Towards Comprehensive Support for Organizational Mining', Decision Support Systems, vol. 46, no. 1, pp. 300–317.

Moon, K.-h. K. (2006). 'Techniques for Designing Case Report Forms in Clinical Trials', ScianNews, vol. 9, no. 1.

Muller-Wilken, S., F. Wienberg and W. Lamersdorf (2000). 'On Integrating Mobile Devices into a Workflow Management Scenario', Paper presented at the 11th International Workshop on Database and Expert Systems Applications (DEXA 2000), 6–8 September.

Santoro, E., E. Nicolis, M. G. Franzosi and G. Tognoni (1999). 'Internet for Clinical Trials: Past, Present, and Future', Controlled Clinical Trials, vol. 19, pp. 194–201.

Seebregts, C. J., M. Zwarenstein, C. Mathews, L. Fairall and A. J. Flisher (2008). 'Handheld Computers for Survey and Trial Data Collection in Resource-Poor Settings: Development and Evaluation of PDACT, a PalmTM Pilot Interviewing System', International Journal of Medical Informatics, vol. 78, pp. 721–31.

Tomlinson, M., W. Solomon, Y. Singh, T. Doherty, M. Chopra, P. Ijumba et al. (2009). 'The Use of Mobile Phones as a Data Collection Tool: A Report from a Household Survey in South Africa', BMC Medical Informatics and Decision Making, 9:51, 23 December.

van der Aalst, W. M. P. (2004). 'Business Process Management Demystified: A Tutorial on Models, Systems and Standards for Workflow Management', in Lectures on Concurrency and Petri Nets: Advances in Petri Nets, edited by Jörg Desel, Wolfgang Reisig and Grzegorz Rozenberg, Eindhoven: Springer, pp. 1–65.

van der Aalst, W. M. P. (2005). 'Business Alignment: Using Process Mining as a Tool for Delta Analysis and Conformance Testing', *Requirements Engineering*, vol. 10, no. 3, pp. 198–211.

van der Aalst, W., T. Weijters and L. Maruster (2004). 'Process Mining, Discovering Workflow Models from Event-Based Data', *IEEE Transactions on Knowledge and Data Engineering*, vol. 16, no. 9, pp. 1041–1142.

van Dongen, B. F., A. K. A. de Medeiros, H. M. W. Verbeek, A. J. M. M. Weijters, W. M. P. van der Aalst (2005). 'The Prom Framework: A New Era in Process Mining Tool Support', in *Applications and Theory of Petri Nets 2005*, edited by Gianfranco Ciardo and Philippe Darondeau, Berlin: Springer, pp. 444–54.

10

A Mobile Electronic Data Capture Solution for Applications in Public Health

Diatha Krishna Sundar, Shashank Garg and Isha Garg

◻

Data collection is an important part of any research study in public health. Traditionally, researchers have used pen-and-paper-based systems for collecting raw data in the field, and this data is then entered into an electronic format database by others, who may not have been involved in primary data collection. Transcribing data from paper to computer format is inherently error-prone, since the transcribers are far removed from the raw data collection process. It is expensive and time-consuming to go back to the field force for problems in the field data. Errors in data collection may result in duplication and unreliable data, which may then result in expensive data cleaning steps being applied, thereby increasing costs and latency in the system. The cost of correcting for errors is lowest when errors are detected at the source of input itself, and this cost increases progressively as data moves within the system further away from the source. Further, longitudinal studies, which require periodic follow-up of a cohort, pose additional challenges due to their long-term nature. Pen-and-paper-based studies are also not easily scalable and replicable. While electronic data capture (EDC) systems have become popular in recent times with the advent of low-cost mobile devices, most EDC systems are proprietary and not easily customisable. In this chapter, we present a generic and flexible EDC solution which is based on open standards that enable the solution to be deployed on a variety of mobile devices.

Field data collection poses many challenges to researchers and practitioners in public health due to many reasons, such as geographical dispersion of the target population, problems of coordination of the field force and the participating subjects, errors in data collection, timely transmission of data, scalability, and follow-up in the case of longitudinal cohort studies. Traditionally, paper-based questionnaires have been used to collect patient data, involving a process which is labour-intensive, time-consuming, error-prone and costly, since data has to be transcribed from paper to electronic format before it can be analysed (Bart 2003; Walther et al. 2011). The process of data collection requires many activities, such as field visits for interviewing subjects, transcription from paper to electronic format, data cleaning and data coding, all of which are potential sources of error (Galliher et al. 2008).

Several comparative studies have been carried out for comparing the effectiveness of EDC systems with paper-based surveys (Bart 2003; Bushnell et al. 2003; Galliher et al. 2008; Walther et al. 2011). Electronic data capture systems can help reduce errors by providing an electronic audit during the process of data collection, as well as help in the monitoring and tracking of subjects during various phases of the study (Turner et al. 2011). Electronic data capture systems also provide a structured procedure for data collection, which is difficult to follow with paper-based surveys as the size of a registry or the size of a cohort in a research study increases. While paper-based case report forms (CRF), or even simple spreadsheets, have been used for data collection in clinical practice settings, these solutions are not inherently suitable for large registries because they are not secure or scalable, and not easily accessible to geographically dispersed users (Shah et al. 2010). Electronic data capture systems are now available for a variety of mobile devices with different form-factors such as personal digital assistants (PDAs), tablets and digitiser pens. Several comparative studies have been done on the usability of these systems in public health research (Cole et al. 2006; Singleton et al. 2011; Walther et al. 2011). Though EDC systems have been deployed in a variety of healthcare settings (Bellamy et al. 2009; Bushnell et al. 2003; Cole et al. 2006; Dykes et al. 2006; El Emam et al. 2009; Gurland et al. 2010; Marks 2004; Pace and Staton 2005; Wilhelm et al. 2006), their general applicability remains limited. Web-based EDC tools, like Lime Survey, SurveyMonkey and SurveyGizmo, and OpenClinica have proved popular, but such systems often have limitations, since internet connectivity may not be available in the field (Singleton et al. 2011). REDCap is another flexible EDC solution, which uses metadata and workflow-based methodology, and

delivers web-based forms for deployment in clinical and translational research (Harris et al. 2009). There are several data collection
projects that are derived from the Open Data Kit, a set of free and
open-source tools for authoring electronic forms, collecting data in
the field, and managing mobile data collection solutions. Open Data
Kit Collect is built on the OpenROSA specification, a subset of the
XForms standard designed for cell-phone-based data collection (ODK
2012; OpenROSA 2012). Another free and open-source platform for
electronic data collection that uses XForms technology extensively
is OpenXdata, with which one of the authors of this chapter has
been associated since its inception. This project was funded by the
Research Council of Norway through the Center for International
Health at the University of Bergen, Norway (OpenXdata 2011).

While a comprehensive set of commercial as well as open-source
EDC tools are now available, adoption of EDC techniques by public
health researchers has been slow due to reasons such as network
constraints and costs, the relative maturity of tool vendors in a new
space, and due to study designers and administrators being risk-
averse (Shah et al. 2010). A comparative study was done on data
collection methods using a range of mobile devices such as PDAs,
tablets, digitiser pens and other digitiser methods for data collection
in clinical trials, in which the digital pen was established as the most
convenient (Cole et al. 2006).

There are many advantages of organising data. It is much easier
if it resides in a database where the data can be more easily manipu-
lated. Analytic tools can import data from a variety of sources such as
spreadsheets and database tables. This implies that a study designer
also has to design the database schema to enable data to be stored in
the database. Longitudinal studies impose additional requirements
on the study designer and implementers, which add to the already
insurmountable list of problems.

The Rationale for an EDC Platform

Research studies in public health often require complex questionnaires to be filled up by fieldworkers, and these are usually in
pen-and-paper format. The traditional fieldworker asks questions
of the respondent and enters responses in a paper questionnaire.
At the end of a field visit, this data is transcribed from paper into
a spreadsheet or database, which is subsequently used for analysis

of the data. Pen-and-paper-based data collection methods have several problems, such as error-prone data collection, errors during transcription and lack of scalability when the size of the respondent population increases.

Since such longitudinal studies require periodic follow-up visits, baseline data has to be maintained and can undergo other changes. Additional questions may be added to the baseline questionnaires or new questionnaires may be required. If additional questions are added to a previous questionnaire, version management becomes a significant issue. If new questionnaires are added, in many cases, baseline data has to be copied into the new questionnaires. Therefore, a form or questionnaire may have many versions being used simultaneously. All of these requirements pose problems that public health professionals and researchers are not technically equipped to handle.

While EDC tools have been around for many years, the advent of mobile technologies, such as smartphones and wireless tablets, now makes it possible to use these mobile devices for a variety of complex surveys. Mobile technologies can play a critical role in assisting healthcare researchers and providers in delivering timely medical response to local clusters of disease and in containing the outbreaks. A wireless-enabled mobile device provides the ideal platform for collection of data in the field which is accurate and validated, and then for transmitting it to a centralised location for analysis and feedback in real time. It empowers the field health-worker to travel to remote areas for data collection and report information in real time, and help the epidemiological community increase health coverage to under-served remote communities.

In this chapter, the authors present eCollect, a mobile EDC solution with which they have been associated during its development and implementation. The eCollect EDC system is a generic and flexible mobile solution based on open standards like XForms, an open specification for electronic forms that is designed to enable platform independence (Boyer 2009).

The focus of this chapter is on providing an overview of the technologies used in this solution, and the enhancements made in eCollect, with reference to a few practical examples. The mobile EDC system presented here is currently being used in many longitudinal studies in public health research, and the ongoing challenges, learning and experiences with different mobile devices will subsequently be published, so that other researchers and practitioners in public health, technology professionals developing practical mobile solutions, and policy experts can be made aware of such mobile solutions.

XForms Technology

Electronic forms which are used for all interactions between different user entities in an EDC system are based on XForms technology that provides a separation between form design and form rendering, such that a form is not specifically tied to any specific platform (Boyer 2009). This platform independence enables different users to choose a mobile device that is most appropriate to their needs, or even support multiple mobile devices, if required. The XForms specification is an open standard that uses a *model-view-controller* approach to enable the design of electronic forms. The *model* provides the essential constructs for handling form data; the *view* describes the way user interface (UI) controls would appear on a form; the *controller* orchestrates all data manipulations and the interactions between the *model* and *view* layers, as well as data submissions to a server. XForms provides support for multiple data types, field validation logic and skip rules, to define the flow of input based on specified conditions. These features, when embedded in an electronic form, provide a technology framework that helps in minimising errors at the source of input.

An XForms engine is essentially an interpreter that interprets the XForms syntax and metadata to carry out the intent of an XForms document and can be implemented on any mobile device. The separation between form definition and form rendering enables different mobile devices to render an electronic form differently but still perform the same set of functions for data collection. An electronic form may contain complex validation rules, skip logic and computations embedded within the form metadata, and the interpreter is able to implement the intent of these built-in functions. Contemporary web browsers already incorporate an XForms rendering engine and are therefore capable of rendering XForms on a web page. Mobile clients have also been implemented for low-cost Java-enabled cell phones.

Some of the benefits of using the XForms approach to developing electronic forms in any application that requires data collection or user input are:

1. Rich set of field data types

   a. Fields can have many data types such as alpha, numeric, decimal, date, global positioning system (GPS), image, audio, video, etc.

2. Field-level validation

   a. Field validation rules can be applied to any input field in a form to validate the data while it is being entered, to prevent erroneous or nonsensical values from being accepted at the source of input itself.
   b. Fields can have range checks.

3. Fields can have calculations based on values in other previously filled fields
4. Flow of questions can be changed.

   a. Complex skip logic rules can be used to change the sequence of questions based on field values in previously filled fields.

5. Separation between form and function is useful in designing UIs for mobile applications.
6. Platform independence

The platform independence that is made possible by using XForms-compliant electronic forms allows different mobile devices to render the form differently and yet perform the same set of functions for data collection. Since XForms has many rich features, some of which were just listed, the adoption of XForms technology provides a level of platform and device independence that will enable solution providers and open-source communities to invest in the development of tools using the standard specifications.

This is already evidenced by the availability of many open-source EDC tools and frameworks, such as OpenXdata, OpenClinica and OpenRosa, which are based on XForms technology for electronic forms. Though these projects initially started out as stand-alone initiatives focusing on specific application areas in public health, there is now a concerted move in each of these developer communities to develop interfaces that will enable data exchange across these diverse systems through the use of XForms technology. This will enable researchers to use the tools that are most appropriate to a specific requirement with the confidence that data can be exchanged seamlessly across these disparate systems when required.

Architecture of the eCollect EDC System

The eCollect mobile EDC system is primarily based on the OpenXdata platform, an open-source community developed platform with which one of the authors of this chapter has been closely associated since its inception (OpenXdata 2011). While the core of eCollect is based on the OpenXdata platform, the eCollect developers have made significant enhancements to the platform in response to specific user needs. Significant enhancements have occurred in the mobile client application, workflows, support for short messaging service (SMS) alerts, enhancements to electronic forms, and in other areas.

The eCollect application server comprises a persistent database, and a set of servelet components that manage the design of studies and forms, the download of studies and forms, uploading of data from mobile clients, and a scheduler for performing several administrative tasks such as export of data from forms, which are basically XML documents containing data encapsulated in unique field tags, to tables with the same names as the unique field tags in the persistent storage. The eCollect server comprises a software stack hosted on a Tomcat servelet container and a MySQL database server.

The architecture of the eCollect system which comprises many software components is shown in Figure 10.1.

Server administration is provided through a web-based dashboard application that manages all the administrative tasks relating to the creation of users on the server, assigning roles and permissions to users, scheduling of activities, and export of data to the persistent database, etc. The server's functionality can be enhanced by developing additional functionality through servelet components which can then be embedded within the server or through an independent servelet which is loosely coupled to the server. This is particularly relevant when the eCollect architecture must interwork with other enterprise applications through web services interfaces. In fact, this is already being done by a development team under the guidance of one of the authors to implement a mobile platform, with a flexible and open architecture, for deployment of mobile governance applications using the eCollect system but customised to governance-specific requirements.

Figure 10.1   Architecture of eCollect, a mobile EDC system

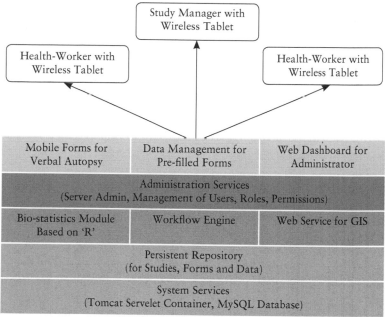

Source: Prepared by the authors.

The Forms Designer is a web-based software component of eCollect that is used to remotely design electronic forms. The Forms Designer implements a subset of the XForms specification to improve the quality of the data collection process at the source of data itself. Features such as field validation rules, range checks, date fields, inter-field calculations, complex skip logic for question sequencing, etc., are all available. All these features help improve the quality of data and avoid the need for double entry. Field data types that are supported are text, alphanumeric, numeric, decimal, Boolean, date, time, date and time, single select, single select dynamic, multiple select, GPS, as well as audio, video and images. Assignment of specific codes to each of the optional data values is permitted in every field that can have multiple options to choose from, including the default values. This helps to eliminate a specific coding step that is often required in traditional data collection systems. Another useful feature of the Forms Designer is that the schema for the database tables is automatically designed during the process of forms design, thereby eliminating an important database design step in traditional approaches.

In addition to the standard data types already supported in OpenXdata's implementation of the Forms Designer, the eCollect system has enhanced the capabilities of the Forms Designer further. A field data type called 'Scribble' is provided to capture 'electronic ink', in an electronic form, using a pen-stylus, if the mobile device supports a touch and pen interface. The scribble feature is very useful for capturing a signature on a form, or for capturing a handwritten narrative in any language. Another field data type for 'text area' with full HTML editing capability is also available. This field data type is further enhanced to support transliteration so that text can be written in a user-selectable local Indian language using an appropriate phonetic keyboard.

The Forms Designer also provides an option to export a form to an XML file for archival storage, and an import function to import a previously exported XML file. The Forms Designer performs several important tasks such as maintaining consistency of form definitions, form layout, binding of variables, managing JavaScript, managing different versions of forms and organising forms under a study hierarchy. Since all electronic forms in the eCollect system are based on XForms technology, support for rendering forms on different mobile devices is provided through a set of mobile client applications on a few popular mobile devices, such as low-cost Java-enabled cell phones, Android-based smartphones and wireless tablets.

A mobile client application provides the primary access mechanism for a health-worker or field data collector to interact with the eCollect data collection system. A mobile client application is essentially an XForms interpreter which can be developed virtually for any device, to leverage the specific capabilities of that mobile device. While any electronic forms designed using the Forms Designer can be rendered using a device-specific XForms interpreter to implement the functionality defined in the XForms metadata, the actual look and feel of the form may be implemented differently on each mobile device based on the graphic and other capabilities of the mobile device. This device-specific interpreter approach allows the XForms to work across a range of mobile devices in a device-independent manner.

The mForms client application, directly derived from OpenXdata's mobile client application, is designed to run on any low-cost Java-enabled mobile device. Since cell phones typically have a small screen which does not have the display capabilities of a regular notebook, the UI on the cell phone is quite different from that of a mobile client designed for a notebook. The mForms client does not support the layout features of an electronic form and instead supports a linear display of questions, which presents the questions in a vertically scrolling format. This independence from the underlying hardware and software operating environment within mForms using the XForms approach provides a unique, ubiquitous capability, since device characteristics are not a limiting factor in using electronic forms on different types of mobile phones. Figure 10.2 shows the flow of an electronic form in the system from the perspective of the mobile user.

Figure 10.2   The Flow of an Electronic Form

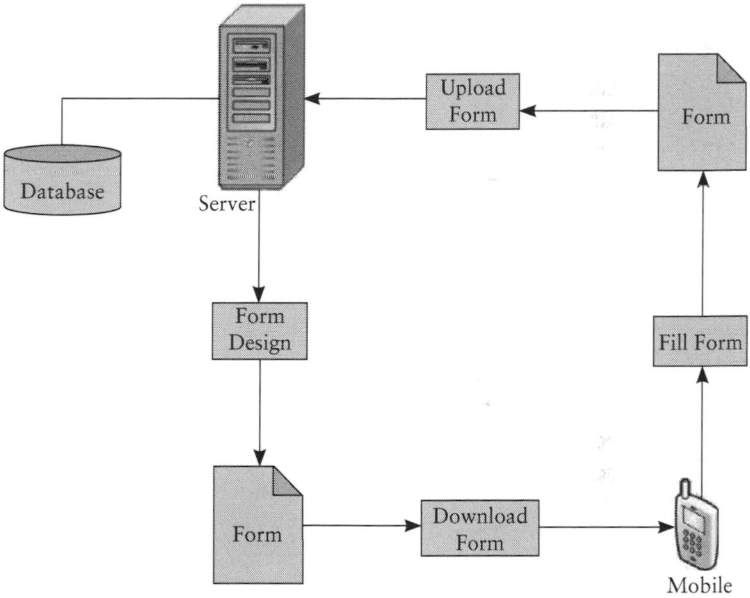

Source: OpenXdata (2011).

Once a form has been designed and published to the server (using the web-based Forms Designer tool), it is available for downloading to a cell phone after it has been mapped to a specific user. When raw data is collected and sent from the mobile device to the server, it is stored in XML form on the server for use by any application that understands the XML format. The collected XML data is also automatically exported to persistent storage in the database from where other applications can access that data; it can also be exported to a CSV file for exchange with other applications.

While the OpenXdata community has developed an mForms client that runs on any low-cost cell phone and is available as a standard feature in OpenXdata, a more feature-rich client application called eCollect is now available as an alternative on the eCollect system. The eCollect application has been developed by one of the authors of this chapter. The eCollect client application interprets XForm metadata within the environment of an HTML5-compliant web browser, thereby making it possible to use this application on any platform that supports an HTML5-compliant web browser.

A common theme between mForms and eCollect clients is their ability to work in a *disconnected* or *offline* mode. Connectivity to the server is only required when downloading forms from the server to the mobile device and when uploading data to the server from the mobile device. This *disconnected mode* of operation enables mobile fieldworkers to work in remote areas for extended periods of time where cellular or other forms of connectivity may not always be available or reliable.

The eCollect client application has many other enhancements and features that are not available in mForms, primarily because it works on mobile devices with rich graphical interfaces and the larger display form-factor of such mobile devices as wireless tablets and smartphones, compared to the lower form-factor of the ordinary J2ME-enabled cell phone. For example, the major difference between the mForms client and the eCollect client is in the handling of layout information embedded within the XForms metadata in a form. The eCollect client is able to use layout information to present information in a way that is closest to a well-designed paper questionnaire, whereas mForms uses no layout information but presents questions in a vertically scrolling linear format. Another enhancement in eCollect is the support for Java-scripting, a feature that can be deployed in complex forms to implement functionality not easily implemented within the existing data types and controls provided by the XForms interpreter. This client-side Java-scripting enables forms to implement complex functions which may not be available in the basic set of XForms validation rules.

Other enhancements such as a rudimentary guidance system for health-workers and online help have been provided through the concept of a 'cheat sheet', an XML document which presents information in the form of a tree structure designed to guide health-workers by prompting them to ask additional relevant questions that may be required.

The different mobile clients have their specific niche uses. A major advantage of the mForms client is its ability to work on any low-cost cell phone that provides a Java virtual machine (J2ME environment) in a small memory footprint, but its main limitation is that it cannot leverage all the features available in the XForms specification without increasing the memory footprint and thereby deviating from the principle of low cost. On the other hand, mForms is relatively easy to learn. So, mForms would be useful in budget-constrained applications where fieldworkers may not have exposure to advanced mobile devices.

A major advantage of a browser-based client application is its ability to operate across different operating environments and hardware platforms, which was the original intent of XForms technology. Thus, the eCollect client can run on any Android smartphone or wireless tablet. The development of the eCollect client application was motivated and driven primarily by the needs of public health researchers in India, who prefer to use larger-format mobile devices than their counterparts in other parts of the world.

A special version of the HTML5 browser-based client application is called mCollect, which runs on an Android smartphone and connects to the eCollect server for access to forms and uploading of data. With the availability of mForms and mCollect client applications, it is now possible to provide users a choice of devices for data collection.

Workflow Management

The eCollect EDC system incorporates a workflow engine based on YAWL, an open-source framework and workflow definition language, capable of capturing all sorts of flow dependencies between tasks (YAWL 2011). It incorporates a graphical editor with built-in verification functionality, which helps in the design of workflow processes and sharing of information between processes through forms. A workflow provides an abstraction for the definition, execution and automation of business processes where tasks, information or documents are passed from one actor to another for action in accordance with a set of procedural rules (Aalst and Hee 2009). A typical workflow consists of a sequence of connected steps to be followed towards achieving an objective. To define a workflow, one needs to specify the tasks that will be executed, the sequence of tasks, the resources for each task, and how tasks are to be mapped to the resources. In order to determine the routing of tasks, workflows require that some data be available to enable decision making. This is implemented in the eCollect platform using pre-filled forms.

Components of the workflow system include a workflow engine, administration interface, process definition interface (workflow editor) and a set of services that are invoked when a task is enabled. The workflow engine ensures that schedules for task execution are adhered to and the relevant data is passed from one task to another. The actual execution of tasks is done through services. The engine is based on a service-oriented architecture where services are registered and called based on a predefined process model. The word 'service', in this case, refers to a set of related software functionalities, together with the policies that control its usage.

A unique feature of mForms and eCollect, the two different mobile client applications described in this chapter, is their ability to operate in offline or disconnected mode, so that a mobile user can collect data in the field without requiring connectivity to a back-end server, once the appropriate set of electronic forms have been downloaded to the mobile phone. The offline client application (mForms or eCollect) handles all the layout information embedded within the form itself which has been downloaded to the mobile device and renders it on the mobile device using device-specific capabilities. Both client applications have function control buttons for download of forms from a remote server, uploading of data and several other maintenance tasks. Once a form is downloaded to the mobile device, along with all its related resources, connectivity is no longer required even though a web interface is used for collection of data. Data collected through locally resident electronic forms is stored in a local object store till it can be uploaded to the back-end server.

The workflow management tool is a simple way to specify and control processes involving field data collection and other tasks for a given application. The system provides the functionality to control workflow items on mobile devices even when the mobile devices operate in disconnected mode, i.e., asynchronously. This is possible because during synchronisation with the application server, the scheduled workflow items are downloaded to the mobile device for data collection, or data for completed workflow items is automatically uploaded to the application server and passed on to the workflow engine for further processing. Hence, the mobile client application supports workflow-based data collection through the process of synchronisation of workflows between the mobile device and the workflow engine running on the remote back-end server. This is an important feature since data collection is just one aspect of an EDC system. Workflows are also required in a comprehensive EDC system because data collection comprises a set of tasks to be executed in a specific sequence which can easily be defined through workflows.

Hence, even though the mobile client may operate in offline mode, at the time of synchronisation with the server, the workflow engine ensures that only the workflow items assigned to that user are downloadable, so that the user can perform only those tasks that have been assigned to him. The workflow engine also provides alerts through email or SMS so that the recipient can log into the server and reclaim the next workflow assigned to that user. This enables the user to stay in sync with the workflow system, without being required to be continuously online.

Analytics Tools

Every research study that requires a data collection system has a specific set of objectives, either to make some inferences, or to prove/disprove/test a hypothesis, or to measure some parameters. Thus, data collection has to be followed up with careful analysis of the data. The Analyzer is essentially a tool integrated into the eCollect forms-based data collection package, so that data collected through mobile phones can be seamlessly analysed. The Analyzer is also generic enough that it can be used as a general-purpose analysis tool for practically any kind of data. Data can be imported from a variety of sources such as CSV formats, spreadsheets, databases, text files, SPSS data files, etc., for subsequent analysis. The Analyzer uses the powerful open-source statistical language called 'R' for its back-end work (R-project 2011). The results obtained are dependable and can be cited in research papers, and will find acceptance everywhere, particularly because of the growing popularity of R in the field of statistics amongst academic and industrial researchers. While R is essentially a command-driven language, the Analyzer provides an enhanced, easy-to-use, SPSS-like UI, to make it convenient for beginners and experts to get their job done without having to memorise all R commands. The power users, whose needs cannot be fulfilled by the UI and who need more control over their analysis, can directly type R commands inside the UI as the Analyzer exposes the full power of R through a console window. The Analyzer also has documentation features built into it, which are very useful for documentation of research. With this feature, R commands can be stored for reference with their results in a separate output window. This helps in reproducibility, an essential feature that is helpful in citing results in research papers and for others to verify and reproduce the results.

Data Management Tools

This is a set of tools for managing data after it has been collected on the server. This combination of tools is used to create cohorts for further follow-up, longitudinal studies, etc. The data management tools comprise a powerful Query Builder and Data Mapper in a single application. It enables a study manager to search collected data using a simple application and to create partitioned data sets. Inclusion and exclusion criteria, which are essential for the analysis of large data sets, can be specified through simple Boolean rules, and complex queries can be built without any knowledge of Structured Query Language, using the Query Builder functionality. The data that satisfies the search criteria can be assigned to specific data collectors. This job is done by a tool called the Data Mapper. When a data collector logs in through the offline client and clicks on 'Download Data', she would be assigned these pre-filled forms that have been mapped to her. This is the type of task typically required for follow-up visits. The data management tools also enable the study manager to copy data from one form to another form or from an external source like a database table or a spreadsheet to a form. These data management capabilities are often required for longitudinal studies.

Geographical Information System Tools

A core set of geographical information system (GIS) tools is also available on the eCollect electronic data collection platform to enable researchers and users to visualise their data on maps. A variety of GIS data-interchange formats are supported so that shape files can be imported from many other web sources. Thus, a shape file can be imported from other online resources and rendered on a blank map. The GIS interface provides a powerful search facility to enable users to partition data into data sets and view it on a selected map. This interface is closely tied to the forms interface, since field data is organised in the database through the schema that was defined during the forms design stage. A GIS user can click on a particular icon on the map to view the consolidated data relating to a particular point in real time, as it is extracted from the database. Advanced features such as choropleths are also provided for present data, in different colours, to represent the density of a particular attribute in the selected map. Multiple layers can be added to the map to store user-specified attributes, and layers can be selected or deselected as required. If the data is collected on a mobile device with GPS, then the location information is used to plot the map on the underlying shape file. Thus, the GIS tools provide a powerful visual aid in the spatial analysis of data.

Discussion and Conclusion

Electronic data capture tools have become essential in the portfolio of public health researchers because of their ability to overcome the shortcomings of traditional pen-and-paper-based systems which are inherently error-prone and not scalable as the size of a study increases.

The lack of standardisation, the propensity amongst public health researchers to be risk-averse, and the lack of domain knowledge amongst solution providers has prevented the large-scale adoption of EDCs. However, the advent of open standards such as XForms for the implementation of electronic forms that are device-agnostic, and HTML5-compliant web browsers capable of supporting disconnected or offline mode of operation, has helped popularise many projects that have leveraged these standards. One such mobile solution, the eCollect EDC system presented in this chapter, has been deployed successfully in many public health research studies.

Web-based EDC solutions are popular with study managers and researchers in public health because they run within a web browser and do not require any additional software to be installed locally. But web forms are often not the ideal solution in field scenarios because of poor internet connectivity when health-workers go into the field (Singleton et al. 2011). However, the eCollect solution presented in this chapter is based on web forms which use a unique approach in which the client application runs within the context of a web browser, but is also able to operate in disconnected or offline mode. It incorporates an XForms interpreter to render electronic forms on any mobile device that uses an HTML5-compliant web browser. The HTML5 standard specification enables offline access to a web page by downloading and locally storing all the resources embedded within a page. Since the mobile client application has to handle several complex objects, the eCollect offline client implements a local object store which saves all the embedded objects of the mobile form within the object store. Hence, the client application can stay disconnected for long periods of time, and only requires connectivity to download mobile forms and to upload data. Thus, the data collector uses a web form to fill out a form, and yet does not have to worry about internet connectivity in the field. A major benefit of this approach is that this mobile client application can run on virtually any mobile device, including a smartphone that has a web browser.

The eCollect EDC system presented in this chapter is built on several open standards such as XForms and HTML5, and incorporates a comprehensive set of capabilities to meet the requirements of researchers and practitioners in public health. These tools can be used to build specific applications that may be required in public health.

—

References

Aalst, W. V. D., and K. V. Hee (2009). *Workflow Management: Models, Methods and Systems*, Cambridge, MA: MIT Press.

Bart, T. (2003). 'Comparison of Electronic Data Capture with Paper Data Collection', *Business Brieûng: Pharmatech*, http://www.dreamslab.it/media/docs/eclinica[1].pdf (accessed on 7 February 2015).

Bellamy, N., C. Wilson, J. Hendrikz, B. Patel and S. Dennison (2009). 'Electronic Data Capture (EDC) Using Cellular Technology: Implications for Clinical Trials and Practice, and Preliminary Experience with the m-Womac Index in Hip and Knee OA Patients', *Inflammopharmacology*, vol. 17, no. 2, pp. 93–99.

Boyer, J. M. (2009). XForms 1.1, W3C Consortium, http://www.w3.org/TR/2009/REC-xforms-20091020/ (accessed on 7 February 2015).

Bushnell, D. M., M. L. Martin and B. Parasuraman (2003). 'Electronic versus Paper Questionnaires: A Further Comparison in Persons with Asthma', *Journal of Asthma*, vol. 40, no. 7, pp. 751–62.

Cole, E., E. D. Pisano, G. J. Clary, D. Zeng, M. Koomen, C. M. Kuzmiak, B. K. Seo, Y. Lee and D. Pavic (2006). 'A Comparative Study of Mobile Electronic Data Entry Systems for Clinical Trials Data Collection', *International Journal of Medical Informatics*, vol. 75, nos 10–11, pp. 722–29.

Dykes, P. C., A. Benoit, F. Chang, J. Gallagher, Q. Li, C. Spurr, E. J. McGrath, S. M. Kilroy and M. Prater (2006). 'The Feasibility of Digital Pen and Paper Technology for Vital Sign Data Capture in Acute Care Settings', *AMIA Annual Symposium Proceedings*, pp. 229–33.

El Emam, K., E. Jonker, M. Sampson, K. Krleza-Jeriæ and A. Neisa (2009). 'The Use of Electronic Data Capture Tools in Clinical Trials: Web-Survey of 259 Canadian Trials', *Journal of Medical Internet Research*, vol. 11, no. 1, p. e8.

Galliher, J. M., T. V. Stewart, P. K. Pathak, J. J. Werner, L. M. Dickinson and J. M. Hickner (2008). 'Data Collection Outcomes Comparing Paper Forms with PDA Forms in an Office-Based Patient Survey', *Annals of Family Medicine*, vol. 6, no. 2, pp. 154–60.

Gurland, B., P. C. Alves-Ferreira, T. Sobol and R. P. Kiran (2010). 'Using Technology to Improve Data Capture and Integration of Patient-Reported Outcomes into Clinical Care: Pilot Results in a Busy Colorectal Unit', *Diseases of the Colon and Rectum*, vol. 53, no. 8, pp. 1168–75.

Harris, P. A., R. Taylor, R. Thielke, J. Payne, N. Gonzalez and J. G. Conde (2009). 'Research Electronic Data Capture (REDCap) — A Metadata-Driven Methodology and Workflow Process for Providing Translational Research Informatics Support', *Journal of Biomedical Informatics*, vol. 42, no. 2, pp. 377–81.

Marks, R. G. (2004). 'Validating Electronic Source Data in Clinical Trials', *Controlled Clinical Trials*, vol. 25, no. 5, pp. 437–44.

ODK (2012). Open Data Kit, http://opendatakit.org/ (accessed on 7 February 2015).

OpenROSA (2012). The OpenROSA Consortium, http://www.dimagi.com/collaborate/openrosa/ (accessed on 19 February 2015).

OpenXdata (2011). Open-Source Software for Data Collection, http//www.openxdata.org (accessed on 7 February 2015).

Pace, W. D., and E. W. Staton (2005). 'Electronic Data Collection Options for Practice-Based Research Networks', *Annals of Family Medicine*, vol. 3, suppl. 1, pp. S21–S29.

R-project (2011). The R Project for Statistical Computing, http://www.r-project.org/ (accessed on 7 February 2015).

Shah, J., D. Rajgor, S. Pradhan, M. McCready, A. Zaveri and R. Pietrobon (2010). 'Electronic Data Capture for Registries and Clinical Trials in Orthopedic Surgery: Open Source versus Commercial Systems', *Clinical Orthopaedics and Related Research*, vol. 468, no. 10, pp. 2664–71.

Singleton, K. W., M. Lan, C. Arnold, M. Vahidi, L. Arangua, L. Gelberg and A. A. Bui (2011). 'Wireless Data Collection of Self-Administered Surveys Using Tablet Computers', *AMIA Annual Symposium Proceedings*, pp. 1261–69.

Turner, J. A., S. R. Lane, H. J. Bockholt and V. D. Calhoun (2011). 'The Clinical Assessment and Remote Administration Tablet', *Frontiers in Neuroinformatics*, vol. 5, pp. 31–38.

Walther, B., S. Hossin, J. Townend, N. Abernethy, D. Parker et al. (2011). 'Comparison of Electronic Data Capture (EDC) with the Standard Data Capture Method for Clinical Trial Data', *PLoS One*, vol. 6, no. 9, p. e25348, doi:10.1371/journal.pone.0025348.

Wilhelm, F. H., M. C. Pfaltz and P. Grossman (2006). 'Continuous Electronic Data Capture of Physiology, Behavior and Experience in Real Life: Towards Ecological Momentary Assessment of Emotion', *Interacting with Computers*, vol. 18, no. 2, pp. 171–86.

YAWL (2011). 'YAWL: Yet Another Workflow Language', http//www.yawlfoundation.org (accessed on 7 February 2015).

Index

Printed and bound by CPI Group (UK) Ltd, Croydon, CR0 4YY

17/10/2024

01775686-0004